Self-Management for Persistent Pain

Karen Rodham

Self-Management for Persistent Pain

The Blame, Shame and Inflame Game?

palgrave
macmillan

Karen Rodham
Department of Psychology
University of Staffordshire
Stoke-on-Trent, UK

ISBN 978-3-030-48968-7   ISBN 978-3-030-48969-4   (eBook)
https://doi.org/10.1007/978-3-030-48969-4

This Palgrave Pivot imprint is published by the registered company Springer Nature Switzerland AG.
The registered company address is: Gewerbestrasse 11, 6330 Cham, Switzerland

Dedicated to those living with persistent pain, health professionals, researchers and policy-makers. It is my hope that we can work together in collaborment and find a way to make self-management less about the 'self' and more about living well.

ACKNOWLEDGEMENTS

Many people have shaped the ideas in this book. Not all of them will be aware of the impact that they have had on my thinking. I am thinking here of the patients and health professionals with whom I have worked over the years, the snatched conversations with people at professional meetings, the people working in different disciplines who have shown me new ways of looking at things, the people with whom I share an office, the pain team in Brazil whom I was lucky to be able to spend a short time with some years ago. All have greatly shaped my thinking and my practice.

It would be remiss of me not to mention Pete Moore here. He is the designer of the Pain Toolkit. He needs a mention all of his own for his inspirational and tireless work promoting ways to help people manage their pain.

Friends and colleagues have provided me with a useful sounding board when I doubted or lost focus, as well as distraction when I needed to stop and let an idea take shape. Jeff, Paula, Fiona, Povvers, Dempers, DCC, 'The Ladies Wot Lunch club', the 'lone-living-lushes' virtual pub, The Birmingham meet up group: Sue, Liz, Sheila; The Stokie contingent: Tweedy, Ruth, Fiona G, The Temple, David W, Peter K, Burners, Kerry & Phil, Julia la Jupe. And not forgetting Karen, who when she was young (over) filled doughnuts with jam. Thank you one and all.

The Mineral Hospital in Bath (its original building is sadly now in the process of being turned into a posh hotel), and the marvellous team there with whom I worked, taught me much and shaped me as a practitioner. They are an inspirational, warm generous and friendly team who always remember to keep patients front and centre in all they do.

Fellow academics who have done the hard graft of researching pain and publishing their findings into which I have dived, read with interest, learned much from and I hope faithfully represented in this book. And the anonymous reviewers whose words were constructive and made this a better, more coherent piece of work than it otherwise might have been.

Stoke Library as well as the cafes in Emma Bridgewater, Middleport and Spode have provided a haven away from distraction where I can write. Hanley Park, Cauldon Canal and Tittesworth Reservoir gave me somewhere to walk whilst I was pondering difficult ideas and Jubilee2 gave me a place to swim and to think. The monotony of all those lengths gave my brain a break and allowed new ideas to surface.

Family of course are the most important people in my life. And, as only family can be, they are uniquely placed to question me, perhaps more bluntly than friends and colleagues might. They may not know it, but they have kept me grounded throughout the ups and downs that come with putting a book together. They have provided all that was needed: distraction, fun and the reminder to focus on what is important. I appreciate their support through the good times as well as the 'oaty' moments.

And lastly, I would not be a fully fledged crazy cat lady (Rodham 2018a) if I did not recognise the often ill-timed, but always welcome interruptions from my old boys George and Jack. Inheriting them when my lovely Dad died turned out to be one of the most unexpected blessings of my life so far.

INTRODUCTION

This book is about the self-management of persistent pain, and right from the start I want to be very clear that I see pain management as vital. We need pain management as part of our approach to helping people cope with persistent pain. So I am not for one moment saying that pain self-management should be replaced with something else. What I am saying is that I think we need to widen the focus of pain self-management and move away from an almost exclusive emphasis on the self; the person living with pain.

More specifically, this book is about my concern that we have come to rely on self-management as an approach to pain management and have somehow lost focus on the people who live with pain and the context within which they live with their pain. We seem to have forgotten that although self-management is absolutely vital in the process of living well with pain, it is not the only element which is important. So the thesis of this book is that we need to do better at familiarising ourselves with the life-context of those who live with pain, so that when we work with them on suggestions for coping, we do not set them up to fail because their life-context prevents them from implementing our suggestions.

When I first started to think about this issue I had two jobs; I was an academic working in a university and I was also a practising health psychologist working in an NHS pain service. My practice was focused on helping those who were living with Complex Regional Pain Syndrome (CRPS) learn to both cope with their CRPS and find ways of living their lives in spite of their CRPS. Much of my NHS role was focused on pain self-management. It was clear to me that whilst the aims of self-management were incredibly important I felt the emphasis was 'off'. Rather than being the key focus for those living with persistent pain, I thought self-management should be one (albeit very important) part of living well with persistent pain.

Gold standard approaches to pain self-management should include multidisciplinary teams, including for example, physiotherapists, psychologists, nurses, medics and occupational therapists (Faculty of Pain Medicine 2015). Their focus is on one person: the person who lives with persistent pain. However, that person does not live in a vacuum. They live somewhere. Maybe they live somewhere deprived, maybe they live somewhere affluent. Maybe they have good social support. Maybe they have limited or no social support. Maybe they live in an inner city tower block where the lift is often out of order. Maybe they live in a rural area where there is no reliable public transport. Maybe they have high or low health literacy. All of these things (and others) will impact on that person's ability to self-manage.

The longer I worked in the pain field, the more I began to wonder whether there might be another way. But I was plagued by self-doubt. I was worried I was being ridiculously idealistic, unrealistic even. But the more I have read around the subject and talked to health professionals, policy-makers and of course, people who are themselves living with persistent pain, the more I have been inspired by others who have also expressed their concerns. For example, I read the report from the King's Fund authored by Coulter and colleagues (2013) who developed the 'House of Care' model, as well as Dr Robin Youngson's book *Time to Care*. They, and others, have questioned how we do things. I would like to add my voice to theirs.

I fear that we are trapped in a modern day version of 'The Emperor's New Clothes', but we have not yet reached the part of the story where someone shouts: "They are all naked!" Right now, it seems to me that our heads have been turned by metrics; everything has targets, rankings, ratings. Costs must be cut, again and again, even when there is nothing left to be cut. It feels like we are being subjected to Fordist systems of working that were designed for the automated assembly line. Perhaps we would do well to remember that even in assembly lines there is room for subversion. This was detailed in the wonderful paper written by the sociologist Donald Roy that I stumbled upon (and never forgot) during my doctoral studies. The paper was called 'Banana Time' and in it, Roy (1959) documented how assembly line workers broke up the tedium of their days, whilst at the same time ensuring that no one worked too fast or too slow.

I remember sharing my discovery of the Roy paper with Karen, a senior lecturer who later became a dear friend of mine. She mused about a job she had one summer when she was studying; her job was in a factory and she was tasked with putting the jam in jam doughnuts. Her job was very boring. She simply had to push the doughnut onto a metal spike which spurted jam into the doughnut. Every now and then to relieve the boredom, she said that she would push the doughnut onto the spike, not once, but two or three times. She smiled as she was telling me. Well, in truth, she grinned widely as she remembered what it felt like to sit on the assembly line and picture a hapless customer taking a bite out of the overly full doughnut. She always hoped that the doughnut would burst. And even though she would never see the results of her actions, the thought sustained her through the boring shift work. In effect, the workers in the Roy (1959) paper, like my friend, worked out how to play the system to make it work better for them. It seems to me that we need to get better at gaming the health system, or maybe we need to change the game we are playing so that we can make it work better for our patients.

But I digress. The dual focus on improving metrics as well as reducing expenditure in my opinion runs the risk of making us blind to what is important. The health service has become ever more specialised, so much so that it can feel like the whole person is no longer at the centre of the health service. This specialisation has perhaps influenced the way that self-management has developed. It seems to have morphed from something that was originally designed to be a collaborative and supportive endeavour to help a person live well, into something where the sole responsibility lies with the person living with the pain condition to, in effect, manage their symptoms. The very name self-management focuses on the self. It is the individual who is expected to manage and cope with their pain condition. The original collaborative element has fallen by the wayside. A casualty of metricisation?

At this point, it is important again to make very clear that this book IS NOT an attack on self-management. I do not wish to suggest that self-management is unimportant. On the contrary, self-management is vital. There are many places that provide excellent self-management programmes. There are many people working extremely hard to raise awareness of self-management *and* to make self-management accessible. Pete Moore, for example, designer of the Pain Tool Kit, works tirelessly to raise awareness of self-management. Similarly, Pain Concern, a charity for whom I recently co-wrote a leaflet have also worked hard on the self-management front, recently introducing a 'Self-management Navigator Tool' (Pain Concern 2019) designed to help patients and health professionals navigate conversations about self-management. And of course it IS reasonable to expect people to take some responsibility for their health. But in my opinion, self-management is just one part of the puzzle. And I fear that we have forgotten that there are other puzzle pieces of which we should be mindful.

This book is my attempt to dig down the back of the metaphorical sofa and ferret out the other pieces of the puzzle, dust them off and see where they might fit and how they might impact on the individual and their ability to self-manage. These other pieces make up our life context and include financial and social capital, the environment, the economy, the policies imposed by government, the language used when we talk about self-management, the facilities we can or can't access, the ongoing support we can or cannot count on. This book is also my attempt to refocus, to take a wider view of pain self-management. I'd like us to find a different term, one that does not incorporate the word 'self' and the connotations that are tied to that word. I'd like us to continue to include self-management (as I have already said, it is and should be an integral *part* of living well with pain), but I would like us to shift from seeing it as something to aim for towards seeing it as part of a wider approach to living well with persistent pain. I hope that through this book, I can shine a little bit of light on the problem as I see it and in so doing highlight ways in which we might work together to overcome the challenges and find a way to 'do' pain self-management differently.

REFERENCES

Coulter, A., Roberts, S., & Dixon, A. (2013). *Delivering better services for people with long-term-conditions: Building the house of care*. London: The King's Fund.

Faculty of Pain Medicine (2015). Core Standards for Pain Management Services in the UK. Faculty of Pain Medicine, London [https://fpm.ac.uk/standardspublications-workforce/core-standards

Pain Concern. (2019). Self-management navigator tool. Retrieved January 6, 2020, from http://painconcern.org.uk/navigator-tool/

Rodham, K. (2018a). *The making of a crazy cat lady*. Lulu Publishers.

Roy, D. (1959). "Banana Time" Job Satisfaction and Informal Interaction. *Human Organization 18*(4), 158–168.

CONTENTS

CONTENTS

CHAPTER 1

Self-Management: The Panacea for Coping with Persistent Pain?

Abstract In this chapter I explain why I am focusing attention on self-management of persistent pain. I then outline the different definitions of self-management and describe the underlying principles. I explore where the drive for self-management originated and what it was set up to achieve. I then question whether the move towards self-management really is the panacea that it was set up to be for those living with chronic conditions. In short, this chapter sets the scene and the context for the rest of this book.

Keywords Chronic pain • Self-management • Cure • Panacea • Prevalence

For many of us pain is something fleeting which lasts as long as it takes to fix the precipitating illness or injury (think of stubbed toes, broken limbs, toothache and so on). In other words, most of the time pain is something we experience, but know that it will be transient because the thing which caused it is fixable. For increasing numbers of the population though, the experience is very different; pain is an unwelcome visitor who refuses to leave. Indeed, Eccleston et al. (1997: 700) noted that: "In chronic pain, the suffering spills over into all aspects of life. Its senselessness offers a fundamental threat to meaning and identity creating the urge and desire for meaning to be found." Such pain is not fixable. It is long term. Chronic. Persistent. In fact the term 'persistent' is increasingly being used in place of the word 'chronic' to describe long-term pain. The British Pain Society (2013) defines chronic, long-term pain as being

> *pain beyond the time that tissue healing would normally be expected; taken as beyond three months.* (British Pain Society 2013: 6)

So, What Is It Like to Live With Persistent Pain?

Knowing how persistent pain is defined (British Pain Society 2013) is informative but does not tell us what it is like to live with persistent pain. A graphic description of the experience of living with persistent pain was shared in a paper by Chris Eccleston and his team (2013) who described it as being a

> *prolonged experience of an immiserating and disabling disease.* (Eccleston et al. 2013: 59)

The word 'immiserate' was new to me and I had to look it up. It means to make miserable, to impoverish. When you learn that those who live with persistent pain typically have multiple and overlapping problems including anxiety, sleep problems, disability, isolation, reductions in their social and financial capital, loss of job, relationship problems and so on, immiserate seems a very apt word to use. With this in mind, it is perhaps not surprising that the complexity of the persistent pain experience is so testing that it can "teach one about one's own forbearance, resilience, and tolerance of threat" (Eccleston et al. 2013: 59).

So not only is persistent pain very difficult to live with, pain itself is such a hard thing to describe. Words just don't do it justice. This is tricky because persistent pain is often not visible and the only person who knows what the pain is like is the person who is experiencing the pain. As long ago as 1968, McCaffery said that pain is "whatever the experiencing person says it is, existing whenever the experiencing person says it does" (McCaffery 1968: 95). This is an entirely reasonable statement. The trouble is though, that whenever there is something which cannot be objectively measured, as human beings we can be quite suspicious and as a consequence, we do not always trust those who are telling us about it. We might suspect that they are exaggerating, or that they are imagining their pain.

But if we remember the McCaffery quote that pain is whatever the person in pain says it is, surely we should trust the person in pain. However, the slippery nature of trying to work with something as subjective as pain can lead to mistrust. For example, Bernhofer (2011: 1) notes that: "Practitioners who would likely not judge the character of a patient who needs increased amounts of medication to treat hypertension; [...] may believe that a patient whose persistent pain does not respond to standard medications is 'drug-seeking,' a narcotic abuser, or has a current need to 'escape reality'." This speculation has been supported by other researchers exploring the experience of the person living with pain. For example, it has been reported that people living with persistent pain say they have been affected by the attitude of healthcare staff. They may feel that they are being told that their pain is psychological or that they are being labelled as a 'difficult patient'. They struggle with the 'invisibility' of their condition and with the absence of straightforward therapeutic options (Dow et al. 2012).

IF WE CAN'T RELY ON WHAT PEOPLE SAY, HOW THEN DO WE MEASURE PAIN?

Since asking people to describe their pain is not deemed reliable, we have also tried to develop ways of measuring pain objectively. However, the trouble is that measuring such a multifaceted, complex, subjective and internal experience is not straightforward (Williams et al. 2000). This presents us with a perplexing problem, not least because without an accurate valid and reliable measure of chronic pain, we won't know how much pain a person is in and we cannot evaluate the impact and effectiveness of the pain interventions we design.

Typically, 'objective' measures of pain have taken the form of rating scales which invite the patient to rate how bad their pain is on a scale of 1 to 10, where 10 is the worst pain imaginable. At face value, this seems a reasonable question. However, choosing a score to show how bad your pain is, is not as easy as it first sounds. This is because scales are designed to measure pain intensity, but intensity is just one aspect of the pain experience.

Ronald Melzack in a 'think-piece' published in 2005 looked back on the process he went through as he explored new approaches to the way in which pain was described and measured (Melzack and Torgerson 1971).

His work led to the development of the McGill Pain Questionnaire known as the MPQ (Melzack 1975). Sparked by a conversation he had in a pain clinic in the early 1950s with Mrs Hull (someone he described as an "impish, delightful woman in her mid-70s" (Melzack 2005: 201), he took note of how she described the pain she was experiencing following amputation of her diabetic-related gangrenous foot. He noted down the specific words she used. Over time as he met and worked with more and more people living with pain, he added to his list of words. He explored his ideas with lots of other people, all of whom are described in the 2005 think-piece, and eventually identified four key ways of describing pain: sensory, affective, evaluative and miscellaneous. These key elements became the MPQ which remains popular today as a means of measuring pain.

Similarly, decades later, Yorkston et al. (2010) suggested that the chronic pain experience was both multidimensional and individual and as such, they argued that pain rating scales were not likely to be appropriate. They put forward the idea that at least five dimensions needed to be considered when attempting to capture the experience of pain. These included:

- pain intensity (how much it hurts)
- pain quality (type of pain)
- pain location (where it is)
- pain interference (impact on life) and
- temporal aspects (frequency, duration, predictability).

So, if we ask people to rate their pain on a scale from 1 to 10, how do we know what the number they have chosen means? Which of the different pain dimensions is a patient reporting on? Are they scoring the intensity? Or the quality? Or the interference? Or maybe a combination of elements? Existing pain rating scales therefore oversimplify a complex experience, ignore variation in key features of the pain experience (e.g. Clark et al. 2002; Turk and Okifuji 1999; Williams et al. 2000) and mean that we can lose a lot of contextual information (Craig 2009).

In an attempt to further understand the complexity of pain, Kenny et al. (2006: 213) explored whether people had a shared understanding of the meaning of pain descriptors. This is important because "a patient's attempt to communicate pain may not succeed when patient and physician have different languages and frames of reference". Kenny et al. (2006) compared how people from a non-clinical sample used words and numbers to rate pain. They were asked to describe the worst pain they had ever experienced and then to rate this on a Visual Analogue Scale (VAS). They were also asked to create a Verbal Rating Scale (VRS). They were given 15 pain descriptors listed alphabetically. Then they were asked to choose the word they believed described the lowest level of pain and assign it a score of one. They moved through the list of words placing them in order of lowest to highest level of pain until the highest rank of 15 was matched to a corresponding word from the list. Each participant then used the scale they had just developed to rate their own worst pain experience.

Both types of scale (VAS and VRS) are designed and based on the assumption that the people completing the scoring share an understanding of the meaning of the pain descriptors. However Kenny et al. (2006) showed that the way participants used pain descriptors was idiosyncratic. For example, there was little agreement amongst participants as to what each word represented in terms of pain intensity (e.g. 19% chose 'excruciating', 17.6% chose 'very intense' and 12.7% chose 'unbearable'). Using verbal descriptors of pain intensity is therefore not helpful, at least not until or unless agreement can be reached about what each word means. In other words if the medical practitioner and the patient ascribe different meaning to the word descriptor being used to communicate the level of pain being experienced, pain descriptors are not useful in medical consultations.

Similar findings were reported by Hush et al. (2010). In their study, adults with back pain were asked to comment on whether they felt a selection of numerical rating scales captured meaningful changes in their condition. The participants felt that the scales were not fit for purpose because they did not capture relevant functional domains. For example, the participants used the scales to reflect other aspects of their pain experience. One participant said:

For me 'ten' was the pain combined with ... being reliant on other people...as well as coping with the pain. (Sue, 33: 650)

Similarly Jensen et al. (2013) showed that patients with different types of pain (low back pain, fibromyalgia and headache) used different words and phrases to explain their pain. What is not known is whether these pain-quality differences were due to between-group differences in underlying pain physiology, emotional states, pain duration or other, as yet unidentified factors. Indeed, Williams et al. (2000: 457) stated that:

The action of arriving at a rating is better conceptualised as an attempt to construct meaning, influenced by and with reference to a range of internal and external factors and private meanings, rather than as a task of matching a distance or a number to a discrete internal stimulus.

As a consequence, we cannot be sure that these pain scales are measuring the issues that are important to the people who are living with pain, nor do we know whether people who live with pain are using these tools in the way intended by those who developed them; or as expected by the health professionals who use the scales in their practice. In short, pain ratings and pain descriptors are an imperfect measure of pain.

So How Does the Health System Cope with the Problem of Persistent Pain?

Our health system was developed to deal with acute episodic care, not the ongoing supervision, observation and care needed by those living with chronic conditions (Reynolds et al. 2018). Yet the numbers of those living with chronic conditions and therefore needing ongoing health care for these conditions are increasing. And as the numbers needing long-term care and support increase, so too does the cost to the NHS.

Indeed, in 2016, Fayaz and colleagues wrote a paper on the prevalence of persistent pain in the UK. In their introduction they mention that persistent pain has been "highlighted as one of the most prominent causes of disability worldwide" (Fayaz et al. 2016: 1). In terms of how many people are affected by persistent pain, as far as the UK is concerned there is little consensus; Donaldson (2008) estimated that up to 8 million people live with persistent pain. However, eight years later, after they had completed their review of the pain literature, Fayaz et al. (2016) concluded that this was a considerable underestimate. Their review suggested that there were in fact 28 million people in the UK living with persistent pain. This equates to 43.5% of the UK population experiencing persistent pain. Furthermore, when they looked at the data by age, this percentage rose to 62% for those over the age of 75. So, we can see that persistent pain affects a large proportion of the general population, and that as our population ages, the numbers of people affected will increase exponentially.

In addition, a geographical divide in England has also recently been identified. People joke about the north-south divide. I had not realised how much until I made the move from Bath in the south west of the UK to Stoke-on-Trent. Although technically, Stoke is in the Midlands, there was a monotonous regularity of comments about how 'grim' I would find it 'up north'. But, as with many trite phrases, there was perhaps an element of truth, for in a recent paper written by Todd et al. (2018), they not only pointed out that there is a north-south pain divide; they stated that "people in the North of England were more likely to have 'severely limiting' or 'moderately limiting' chronic pain" (Todd et al. 2018: 1). Furthermore, they specifically mentioned that the West Midlands was one of the three areas in England that had the highest prevalence of chronic pain (>40%). This difference in the prevalence and experience of persistent pain is shocking and, as a resident of the West Midlands, and as someone with expertise in the field of persistent pain, I feel a sense of responsibility to do something that will begin to make a difference, not just to the UK, but also for my neighbours here in the Midlands, one of the places with a high prevalence of persistent pain.

It has been said that people with long-term conditions use a disproportionately high level of health and social care services (Potter et al. 2018). This should be seen as a straightforward statement of fact. After all, if you have a long-term condition, of course over time, your needs will be more expensive than someone who has an acute problem which temporarily stops them in their tracks until the problem is fixed and they go on their merry way. However, the word 'disproportionately' can be seen by those living with chronic condition(s) as judgemental. There is, it feels an unnamed amount of time and finance that is considered reasonable for people to use and overstepping that mark (and in so doing, taking more than your fair share) is a 'bad' thing. No wonder people feel judged. Although I am oversimplifying things somewhat here, it can be argued that the combined increase in numbers of people living with chronic conditions has put pressure on a health system that was never set up to deal with chronic conditions. Add to this the years of decreasing investment in our health system, it is not so surprising that a search for a solution has led to the idea that people with chronic conditions *should* (not could, 'should') play a more active role in managing their conditions (Health Foundation 2015; Naylor et al. 2015). For example, Reidy et al. (2016) suggest that self-management is needed to, amongst other things, improve health outcomes, ensure appropriate utilisation of services, increase patient confidence, reduce unplanned admissions, improve adherence to both medicine *and* treatment. Self-management does indeed seem like a cure-all.

SELF-MANAGEMENT AS PANACEA

Self-management as originally intended focused on patients *working with* health professionals. Lorig and Holman (2003) state that Thomas Creer is said to have been the first to suggest that patients should be active participants in their own treatments. Note the wording here is 'participants in' not 'managers of' their treatment. Indeed, the self-management ideal in the healthcare context is that it is something that

> *recognises, harnesses and develops people's assets (empowering and working with them as __partners__ rather than emphasizing their deficits and reinforcing dependency); __support for__ self-management reduces people's needs to health services and thus renders those health services more sustainable; and __support for__ self-management offers people more control over their lives, empowering them and enhancing their well-being as well as their health.* (Morgan et al. 2016: 244 [my emphasis])

The words 'partners' and 'support *for* self-management' here are important. These imply a collaborative, equal relationship where the patient and the health professional work together with mutual respect to find a way to help individuals live well with their long-term condition. This sounds great; helping people to live well with their condition whilst also reducing demands on the creaking health system sounds like the answer we have been looking for. However, before we get too carried away, we need to spend some time thinking about how self-management is defined.

WHAT DOES SELF-MANAGEMENT ACTUALLY MEAN?

'Self-management' itself is an interesting term which is employed in a range of contexts. For example, in the organisational world, Vermeer and Wenting (2016) explain that a self-managing team is one which shares responsibility for achieving goals or results. Since team members are collectively responsible for the team result, each member needs to have a co-operative attitude and a solution-focused outlook. Those who have such attributes avoid getting bogged down in problems and instead find ways to move themselves forward. Self-managing in this context therefore requires a different way of thinking about collaboration. Instead of someone giving orders and monitoring whether or not progress is being made, the team work together to collaborate. They trust one another, communicate well and engage in mutual consultation. To draw from Transactional Analysis, the team members would be considered to be communicating in an 'adult-to-adult' manner (see the classic book by Berne 1964). Clearly this is an ideal and I am sure that many of you reading this now will be more familiar with a more traditional organisational model whereby someone in authority (our line manager) sets our agendas, our tasks, our goals and then watches and monitors us in this metrics-driven world, to make sure we achieve them. The senior person takes on the role of parent, and often, we fall into the role of child. Not so healthy.

The term self-management in the health field is complex and has not proved easy to conceptualise, or indeed, define. For example, Grady and Gough (2014: e26) note that:

> self-management is used widely and is described by a variety of definitions and conceptualisations, which contribute to a lack of clarity and agreement in the literature. At a broad level, self-management is defined as the day-to-day management of chronic conditions by individuals over the course of an illness.

So self-management involves a multitude of actions: managing the condition, engaging in healthy lifestyle behaviours, adjusting to illness enforced changes in our social, vocational, economic roles, making conscious decisions, learning and becoming informed about the condition, forming a good relationship with the health care providers. In short, it is all about taking what are often described as 'appropriate actions'. But who defines appropriate?

Sometimes, behaving appropriately may not be something which is within our control. After all, we are affected by the wider society in which we live, by the systemic, political, economic bigger picture. We are affected by our own financial and social capital, or lack thereof. Yet consistently the self-management definitions focus on the individual whilst ignoring the wider life context. For example, Bringsvor et al. (2018) identified eight domains, all of which are focused on the individual. These include positive and active engagement in life, health directed activities, skill and technique acquisition, constructive attitudes and approaches and health services navigation. Similarly, Nøst et al. (2018: 2) suggest that self-management skills are related to "problem-solving, decision-making, resource utilisation, forming a patient-healthcare provider relationship, and taking action". Padilha and colleagues (2017: 123) note that self-management is itself a dynamic process focusing on the "patient's capacity to self-control the symptoms, the treatment regimen and the physical, emotional and social consequences of the disease". The emphasis is on the patient to make behavioural changes to their daily living habits, to learn to self-monitor their conditions and to ensure they 'implement' cognitive, behavioural and emotional responses needed to control the progression of the disease and of their autonomy and quality of life.

It seems to me that we are expecting a lot from our patients who are learning to cope with their diagnosis, the ramifications of their condition and its impact on all aspects of their life. All of the self-management definitions focus on the individual and we expect patients to quickly become experts so that they do not 'unfairly' use up resources that could be used for others without long-term conditions. Indeed, Packer et al. (2018) note that although many definitions of self-management exist, the definition proposed by the Institute of Medicine (2004) is commonly used:

> *Tasks that individuals must undertake to live well with one or more chronic conditions. These tasks include having the confidence to deal with medical management, role management and emotional management of their conditions.*

This definition, and others, very clearly places the onus on the individual (just look at the word 'must'). Similarly, if we take a look at the coping field, we can see that the dominant approaches for understanding coping almost exclusively focus on the changes (behavioural, cognitive, habitual, physical and emotional) that the individual affected by illness is expected to make (Potter et al. 2018). These changes do not, and in fact, cannot happen in a vacuum. We live in our own life context. Each person's life context will be different. But how we live, and whether we are able to make changes will to some extent be dependent upon, and defined by the social, cultural, financial space in which we live. Furthermore, living with a chronic condition, in other words, a condition that is with us 'for the long haul' does not simply require a one off push to change our ways in order to live with it. The condition may change over time, our life context may change. We age, and with age come other age-related health issues, which in turn could interact with our persistent pain. Each change in turn potentially requires us to alter how we self-manage.

Self-management is therefore dynamic, ongoing, fluid and co-dependent on our wider social, cultural, relational, emotional, financial circumstances. This is an issue highlighted by Borg (2018) in his analysis of themes from Christina Crosby's memoir of her experiences of acquiring a painful, life changing and disabling spinal cord injury. Crosby, a professor of literature, wrote:

> *I am remarkably fortunate that I can continue to do the work I did before I was injured, though I am able to work only half as many hours a week. [...] Nonetheless, with Janet's income added to my reduced paycheck, I still have enough money to be insulated from the indignities of an unjust world in which so many disabled people suffer because their welfare depends on poorly paid personal aides sent out from agencies, public transportation that is often unreliable, and housing that is only barely or not at all accessible.* (Crosby 2016: 5–6)

Crosby is very clear—she has sufficient income because she was able to reduce her hours and keep her job, and her partner was still working. She has social and emotional support from her partner. She is able to afford to pay for the extra help she needs, which means she does not have to rely solely on her partner for intimate self-care activity. This is important, for it helps to prevent the partner's role slipping from partner to carer. Crosby is, as she writes, fortunate. She could self-manage because of the support for self-management she had around her. Crosby did what she could. Of course she self-managed, but this was just one element of her coping strategies. And yet, even though on one hand we know that self-management is fluid and dependent on our life context, self-management as a concept and as a practice in the health service remains firmly focused on the individual and fails to take into account the potential influence of the individual's life context on their ability to self-manage.

How Is Self-Management Measured?

In 2018, two reviews of self-management measures were published. Banerjee and colleagues published the results of a review they had completed of outcome measures designed to assess self-management in patients with chronic pain. Their aim was to identify, appraise and synthesise the range of outcome measures so that they could provide definitive information that would help researchers and clinicians choose the most appropriate tool to assess self-management. In contrast, Packer et al. (2018) focused on two things: one to identify the self-report scales that were being used to measure self-management of adults with chronic conditions and the second to describe the intended purpose, theoretical foundation, scope and dimensionality of the scales.

Both sets of researchers reported that not only were many measures being used, each measure focused on a different aspect of the difficult-to-define-term 'self-management'. Banerjee et al. (2018) identified 14 measures that were used as a proxy measure to assess self-management. In short, a single measure of self-management does not exist, only proxy-measures each assessing a different element of self-management. In addition, although these proxy measures appeared to be well constructed, the age-old call for more research was made so that the reliability and responsiveness of the different measures could be developed. Packer et al. (2018) went further. They identified 28 self-management measures and suggested that since self-management was clearly such a complex, multidimensional construct; what was needed were *new measures* with capacity to quantify and distinguish all aspects of self-management. So both groups identified a plethora of scales in existence, one suggested that more research was needed to make the measures more valid and reliable, whilst the other group called for the development of yet another measure.

To sum up, self-management is measured using questionnaires that have been designed by health professionals and researchers, with little input from people who are themselves living with pain. Since the definition of self-management is diverse, the number of questionnaires purporting either to measure self-management or to act as a proxy measure of self-management is large. As yet, no scale measures self-management in its full multi-dimensional glory. We have measures of self-efficacy, quality of life, psychological well-being, physical functioning, condition-related knowledge, helplessness, emotional support, social support and so on. In short, although there is not a standardised way of measuring self-management, typically the focus of chronic pain self-management encourages individuals to learn how to manage their pain through maintaining their treatment regimen, pacing their activities and learning to control the physical, emotional and social consequences of their condition (Entwistle et al 2018a). Given this complexity, it is unsurprising that its effectiveness has not yet been fully established (Francis et al. 2018).

So, Is Self-Management the Panacea for Coping with Persistent Pain?

It is not clear how all the ideas, factors or underpinning themes that make up self-management hang together. Self-management is something that has been designed by key stakeholders to reduce the demand for limited health care services, to save money and to achieve goals set by professionals, not necessarily goals set by the people who are living with the long-term condition. So, with a cynical head on, one could ask if self-management is really a means of helping the health service cope with persistent pain by shifting responsibility onto the shoulders of those living with pain? It could seem that way.

However, if we return to the coping literature, we do know that "coping is socially negotiated, defined by the social space in which it takes place" (Potter et al. 2018: 131) and that people living with chronic pain need confidence, competence as well as collaborative and supportive relationships with health professionals and significant others (Francis et al. 2018). Indeed, my work with patients, in clinical practice, through research and workshops (e.g. Gauntlett-Gilbert et al. 2015; Navarro et al. 2018; Rodham et al. 2015), shows that people living with persistent pain do not feel that they are being properly equipped or supported to self-manage. For example, patients living with chronic pain who took part in a self-management discussion I ran at a conference in Bath, UK (Rodham 2018) reported that they could not access support to help them manage. They felt that they were left alone to cope and that they were considered to be a burden to the health system and to their family. They said that when they could get appointments with health professionals, these were short and health professionals did not appear to listen to or hear them. Inevitably, this had an impact on how they felt about themselves. One workshop participant said: "It is so hard to self-manage when I hate myself. I don't like who I have become. I am a burden and I don't feel I like myself enough to engage in self-care."

Conclusions

Evidently, self-management, as experienced by people living with pain, is not necessarily positive or empowering. Although self-management is increasingly expected of those living with persistent pain (Entwistle at al. 2018a) the underlying assumptions of self-management programmes fail to consider how, or whether, patients' life context impacts on their ability to engage with self-management. The remainder of this book explores how we might be able to bring life context back to the fore and work towards self-management returning to its roots of being a collaboration rather than an extra burden placed on those individuals already working hard to live well with their persistent pain.

REFERENCES

Banerjee, A., Hendrick, P., Bhattacharjee, P., & Blake, H. (2018). A systematic review of outcome measures utilised to assess self-management in clinical trials in patients with chronic pain. *Patient Education and Counseling, 101*(5), 767–778.

Berne, E. (1964). *Games people play.* New York: Grove Press.

Bernhofer, E. (2011, October 25). Ethics: Ethics and pain management in hospitalized patients. *The Online Journal of Issues in Nursing, 17*(1), 11.

Borg, K. (2018). Narrating disability, trauma and pain: The doing and undoing of self in language. *A Journal of Literary Studies and Linguistics, VIII*, 169–186.

Bringsvor, H. B., Skaug, K., Langeland, E., Oftedal, B. F., Assmuss, J., Gundersen, D., Osborne, R. H., & Bentsen, S. B. (2018). Symptom burden and self-management in persons with chronic obstructive pulmonary disease. *International Journal of COPD, 13*, 365–373.

British Pain Society. (2013). *Guidelines for pain management programmes for adults: An evidence-based review prepared on behalf of the British Pain Society.* London: The British Pain Society.

Clark, W. C., Yang, J. C., Tsui, S. L., Ng, K. F., & Clark, S. B. (2002). Unidimensional pain rating scales: A multidimensional affect and pain survey (MAPS) analysis of what they really measure. *Pain, 98*, 241–247.

Craig, K. D. (2009). The social communication model of pain. *Canadian Psychology, 50*(1), 22–32.

Crosby, C. (2016). *A body undone: Living on after great pain.* New York: New York University Press.

Donaldson, L. (2008). *150 years of the annual report of the Chief Medical Officer: On the state of public health 2018.* London: Department of Health.

Dow, C. M., Roche, P. A., & Ziebland, S. (2012). Talk of frustration in the narratives of people with chronic pain. *Chronic Illness, 8*(3), 176–191.

Eccleston, C., Morley, S. J., & Williams, A. C. d. C. (2013). Psychological approaches to chronic pain management: Evidence and challenges. *British Journal of Anaesthesia, 111*(1), 59–63.

Eccleston, C., Williams, A. C. D. C., & Rogers, W. S. (1997). Patients' and professionals' understandings of the causes of chronic pain: Blame, responsibility and identity protection. *Social Science and Medicine, 45*(5), 699–709.

Entwistle, V. A., Cribb, A., & Owens, J. (2018a). Why health and social care support for people with long-term conditions should be oriented towards enabling them to live well. *Health Care Analysis, 26*, 48–65.

Fayaz, A., Croft, P., Langford, R. M., Donaldson, L. J., & Jones, G. T. (2016). Prevalence of chronic pain in the UK: A systematic review and meta-analysis of population studies. *BMJ Open, 6*, e010364. https://doi.org/10.1136/bmjopen-2015-010364.

Francis, H., Carryer, J., & Wilkinson, J. (2018). Patient expertise: Contested territory in the realm of long-term condition care. *Chronic Illness, 15*(3), 197–209.

Gauntlett-Gilbert, J., Rodham, K., Jordan, A., & Brook, P. (2015). Emergency Department staff attitudes toward people presenting in chronic pain: A qualitative study. *Pain Medicine., 16*(11), 2065–2074.

Grady, P. A., & Gough, R. N. (2014). Self-management: A comprehensive approach to the management of chronic conditions. *Framing Health Matters, 104*(8), e25–e31.

Health Foundation. (2015). *A practical guide to self-management support: Key components for successful implementation.* London: The Health Foundation.

Hush, J. M., Refshauge, K. M., Sullivan, G., De Souza, L., & McCauley, J. H. (2010). Do numerical rating scales and the Roland-Morris disability questionnaire capture changes that are meaningful to patients with persistent back pain? *Clinical Rehabilitation, 24*, 648–657.

Jensen, M. P., Johnson, L. E., Gertz, K. J., Galer, B. S., & Gammaitoni, A. R. (2013). The words patients use to describe chronic pain: Implications for measuring pain quality. *Pain, 154*, 2722–2728.

Kenny, D. T., Trevorrow, T., Heard, R., & Faunce, G. (2006). Communicating pain: Do people share an understanding of the meaning of pain descriptors? *Australian Psychologist, 41*(3), 213–218.

Lorig, K. R., & Holman, H. R. (2003). Self-management education: History, definition, outcomes and mechanisms. *Annals of Behavioral Medicine, 26*(1), 1–7.

McCaffery, M. (1968). *Nursing practice theories related to cognition, bodily pain, and man- environment interactions.* Los Angeles: University of California at Los Angeles Students' Store.

Melzack, R. (1975). The McGill Pain Questionnaire: Major properties and scoring methods. *Pain, 1*, 277–299.

Melzack, R. (2005). The McGill Pain Questionnaire: From description to measurement. *Anesthesiology, 103*, 199–202.

Melzack, R., & Torgerson, W. S. (1971). On the language of pain. *Anesthesiology, 34*, 50–59.

Morgan, H. M., Entwistle, V. A., Cribb, A., Christmas, S., Owens, J., Skea, Z. C., & Watt, I. S. (2016). We need to talk about purpose: A critical interpretive synthesis of health and social care professionals' approaches to self-management for people with long-term conditions. *Health Expectations, 20*, 243–259.

Navarro, K., Wainwright, E., Rodham, K., & Jordan, A. (2018). Parenting people with complex regional pain syndrome: An analysis of the process of parental online communication. *Pain Reports, 3*, e681.

Naylor, C., Imison, C., Smithson, R., Buck, D., Goodwin, N., Ross, S., Sonola, L., Tian, Y., & Curry, N. (2015). Transforming our healthcare system: Ten Priorities for commissioners. Retrieved from https://www.kingsfund.org.uk/publications/articles/transforming-our-health-care-system-ten-priorities-commissioners

Nøst, T. H., Steinsbekk, A., Bratas, O., & Grønning, K. (2018). Short-term effect of a chronic pain self-management intervention delivered by an easily accessible primary healthcare service: A randomised controlled trial. *BMJ Open, 8*, e023017.

Packer, T. L., Fracini, A., Audulv, A., Alizadeh, N., Gaal, B. G. I. V., Warner, G., & Kephart, G. (2018). What we know about the purpose, theoretical foundation, scope and dimensionality of existing self-management measurement tools: A scoping review. *Patient Education and Counseling, 101*(4), 579–595.

Padilha, J. M., Sousa, P. A. F., & Pereira, F. M. S. (2017). Nursing clinical practice changes to improve self-management in chronic obstructive pulmonary disease. *International Nursing Review, 65*(1), 122–130.

Potter, C. M., Kelly, L., Hunter, C., Fitzpatrick, R., & Peters, M. (2018). The context of coping: A qualitative exploration of underlying inequalities that influence health services support for people living with long term conditions. *Sociology of Health & Illness, 40*(1), 130–145.

Reidy, C., Kennedy, A., Pope, C., Ballinger, C., Vassilev, I., & Rogers, A. (2016). Commissioning self-management support for people with long-term conditions: An exploration of commissioning aspirations and processes. *BMJ Open, 6*, e010853.

Reynolds, R., Dennis, S., Hasan, I., Slewa, J., Chen, W., Tian, D., Bobba, S., & Zwar, N. (2018). A systematic review of chronic disease management interventions in primary care. *BMC Family Practice, 19*, 11. https://doi.org/10.1186/s12875-017-0692-3.

Rodham, K. (2018). CRPS and self-management. In *CRPS UK Conference*, October 20, 2018, Bath.

Rodham, K., Gavin, J., Coulson, N., & Watts, L. (2015). Co-creation of information leaflets to meet the support needs of people living with Complex Regional Pain Syndrome (CRPS) through innovative use of wiki technology. *Informatics for Health and Social Care, 41*(3), 325–339.

Todd, A., Akhter, N., Cairns, J. M., Kasim, A., Walton, N., Ellison, A., Chazot, P., Eldabe, S., & Bambra, C. (2018). The pain divide: A cross-sectional analysis of chronic pain prevalence, pain intensity and opioid utilisation in England. *BMJ Open, 8*, e023391. https://doi.org/10.1136/b,jopen-2018-023391.

Turk, D. C., & Okifuji, A. (1999). Psychological factors in chronic pain: Evolution and revolution. *Journal of Consulting and Clinical Psychology, 70*(3), 678–690.

Vermeer, A., & Wenting, B. (2016). *Self-management: How does it work?* Amsterdam: Reed Business Information.

Williams, A. C. D. C., Davies, H. T. O., & Chadury, Y. (2000). Simple pain rating scales hide complex idiosyncratic meanings. *Pain, 85*, 457–463.

Yorkston, K. M., Johnson, K., Boesflug, E., Skala, J., & Amtmann, D. (2010). Communicating about the experience of pain and fatigue in disability. *Quality of Life Research, 19*, 243–251.

CHAPTER 2

Self-Management as Presented in Policy

Abstract In this chapter I address four questions: Who writes self-management policy? How is self-management presented in policy? Who evaluates self-management policy? What is really at the centre of self-management policy? I conclude the chapter with an outline of why I think that self-management policy is flawed.

Keywords Self-management • Policy • Persistent pain • Guidelines

WHO WRITES SELF-MANAGEMENT POLICY?

In the UK, the prime minister is ultimately responsible for all policy and decisions. The prime minister has a cabinet (which is another term for a team) who meet regularly to discuss important decisions. The cabinet is made up of Secretaries of State from all departments and some other ministers. A Secretary of State is a head of a major government department. At the time of writing there are 25 government ministerial departments. The one which is most relevant to this book is currently called the Department of Health and Social Care (at least that is what it is called as I write—politics is fickle and fast changing, so who knows what we will have by the time this book is published!).

It is worth nothing at this point that my work has been based in England and so I am more familiar with and likely to refer to English processes and policies. However, in the spirit of inclusiveness, before returning to the Department of Health and Social Care, I include brief mention here of Scotland, Wales, Ireland and Northern Ireland:

- The Scottish parliament can pass laws on devolved matters that affect day-to-day life in Scotland; these include health. In terms of pain management, NHS Scotland established the Scottish National Residential Pain Management Programme (SNRPMP) in 2015. This has a focus on how the person living with pain can learn new skills to reduce the impact of pain on their life. The pain management programmes involve a three-week residential, followed by a telephone review three months post residential and six months post-residential patients are invited back for a day 'top-up' session.
- Similarly, the National Assembly for Wales is democratically elected and represents the interests of the people of Wales, including holding the Welsh Government to account. The Welsh Government is the devolved government for Wales. In 2019 it published a document setting out aims for how to best help those living with persistent pain.
- The Government of Ireland is made up of 18 departments. The Department of Health is responsible for improving the health and well-being of people in Ireland.
- The Northern Ireland Government is made up of nine departments. The Department of Health has published guidelines (2019) for education programmes and long-term condition self-management.

The stated aim of the Department of Health and Social Care (DHSC) is to support ministers who are leading the nation's health and social care, to help people live more independent, healthier lives for longer. Amongst the DHSC's list of responsibilities are two that are of key relevance to this book. First, the DHSC is responsible for supporting and advising government ministers, and in so doing, the department shapes and delivers the policy that will facilitate delivery of the government's objectives. Second, the DHSC acts as guardian of the health and care framework and makes sure that the legislative, financial, administrative and policy frameworks are fit for purpose. In order to achieve its aims, the DHSC in turn works with 28 agencies and public bodies. These include the National Institute for Health and Care Excellence (otherwise known as NICE) and NHS England.

The relationship between the DHSC and the National Institute for Health and Care Excellence (NICE) is mapped out in the DHSC (2018b) Framework agreement. NICE is described as a national advisory body which has the role of providing "guidance and support to providers and commissioners to help them improve outcomes for people using the NHS, public health and social care services. NICE supports the health and care system by describing what good quality care looks like" (DHSC 2018b: 3). The work NICE engages in is normally set by ministers and NHS England several years in advance. At the time of writing, NICE is developing guidelines for chronic pain, due out in 2020.

NHS England leads the national health service in England. Each year the Secretary of State publishes the objectives and the budget for NHS England. NHS England then leads the commissioning of NHS services in England. The relationship between the DHSC and NHS England is currently set out in the 2019/20 'Accountability Framework' (DHSC 2019). NHS England is currently working towards its most recent plan, known as the 'NHS Long Term Plan', published in January 2019. Self-care and self-management feature in this plan with both being promoted widely. Better support for patients, carers and volunteers to "enhance 'supported self-management' particularly of long-term health conditions" (p33) is also mentioned.

How is Self-Management Presented in Policy?

When you read through the different policies, the stated aspirations of self-management are worthy and difficult to argue with. Self-management (which, incidentally, is rarely explicitly defined) is portrayed as a 'win-win' option: support for self-management gives individuals more control over their lives and at the same time saves the health service money. The ultimate aim is to ensure that people living with long-term conditions are better equipped so that they can go about their daily lives without relying on the health service for anything more than a little collaborative support. As technology gets 'smarter' the intention is to encourage individuals to take on the role of monitoring their symptoms. Individuals are empowered to take responsibility and work with the health profession in partnership. And when this happens, their need for health services is reduced, which in turn means that the services become more sustainable themselves. By way of example, the NHS has recently (January 2019) published its long-term plan, setting out its key ambitions for the service for the next ten years. It made me smile when I read Richard Murray's report about it on the King's Fund website, where he describes the plan thus:

> *The NHS long term plan has been launched and long it indeed is, in every sense of the word: it clocks in at a weighty 120 pages—not including the glossary and references.* (Murray 2019)

Self-management is mentioned as part of the plan to reduce demand for NHS services, although what is meant by 'self-management' is not explained. As such, we cannot be sure what the means for reducing demand are. However we are told that it will be achieved through "improving upstream prevention of avoidable illness and its exacerbations"(NHS 2019: 33). 'Upstream' is another term which is not explained. I can only assume that it refers to the oft told story of the person standing on the banks of the river, pulling out people who are drowning. Eventually the person heads upstream to find out where the drowning people are coming from and learn that a bridge is broken and because of this, people keep falling in. The person fixes the bridge and there are no more drowning people. So I am guessing that the moral of this story is that if we can look upstream and fix the bridge, or in our case "enhance 'supported self-management' particularly of long-term health conditions" (NHS 2019: 33), perhaps we will in turn reduce the demand on the NHS. What is meant by 'supported' as applied to self-management is not explained either. It is a phrase which is only mentioned once in the whole long document. We can therefore assume that this document presupposes that readers will know a) what self-management is and b) what supported self-management looks like. When you consider (as I have already outlined in the previous chapter) that there are many definitions of self-management, this is a problem since without definition, it is not clear what is meant by (supported) self-management in this context.

The Department of Health and Social Care (2018a) recently published their vision to help the UK population live longer, entitled 'Prevention is better than cure'. I read this document with high hopes, which, I am sad to say, were quickly dashed. As with the aforementioned long-term plan there is much in this document that is at face value, very difficult to argue with, for example:

> *our health is one of our nation's most precious and important assets—we must protect and nourish it.* (p5)

action is needed from national and local government to help people make healthier choices. (p19)

However, closer reading of the document shows that the focus is, in the main, on the individual. The first point made in the section on 'preventing problems in the first place' is that "living well starts with individuals and families". Again, this sounds reasonable. But then the focus turns to how decisions we take every day can help us improve our health. These include eating a good diet, being physically active, taking care of our mental health and creating the right home environment to nurture and strengthen our resilience. Again, all reasonable things to say. However, this idealistic view fails to take into account the bigger picture. Living well might start with individuals and families—but only if the context in which they live provides them with the opportunity and ability to choose to live well. The way the document is phrased suggests that living well is a choice. However, for many people living well is not a choice. Living is the priority. Living well is only a choice when you have security in terms of finances, somewhere to call home, a job and so forth. This bigger picture, the 'life context', is invisible in this and other policy documents.

As an aside, I completely understand how easy it is to fall into the trap of being idealistic. I have been known to do it myself. For example, I remember when I moved to Stoke-on-Trent from Bath, I was struck by how many more overweight people seemed to be in Stoke compared to Bath. I also noticed differences in shopping habits; many shopping baskets were full of ready meals with few, if any, fresh ingredients. Once I had settled into life in the Midlands I arranged to talk to a local public health specialist to learn more about Stoke-on-Trent. It is true to say that he opened my eyes. Many people live in accommodation without access to cooking facilities. If they are lucky, they might have a microwave. And even if they do have access to a cooker, they may not be able to afford the cost of using it compared to the cost of the microwave. Ready meals in these circumstances are the sensible option.

Now I do not come from an affluent background; I am one of five children and both my parents worked extremely hard and indeed had more than one job for much of their working lives in order to be able to provide for us. My dad was a teacher all his life, but he supplemented his income at different times by being a taxi driver, a football pools man and a GCSE examiner. My mum was a cleaner in the early hours of the morning for many years which allowed her to be home in time to take us to school. Later, she worked nights in a nursing home to supplement dad's salary and ensure we had enough. We never went without, but we never had an excess. In terms of food, both my parents cooked and made most of our meals from scratch. Not extravagant meals: we had things like stew, shepherd's pie, lasagne, roast dinners, home-made pizza. Most of my friends' parents did the same. So I grew up with some assumptions about food and food preparation. You could call it unconscious bias because I was unaware that for many people, my experiences were far from the norm. And if I was unaware of my biases—how much further removed from the reality experienced by many people struggling to make ends meet are those who set the policies?

So why this diversion into ready meals in Stoke? All this made me think very hard about the assumptions I had been making. Although I thought I was aware of poverty and the problems of living within a tight budget, my experience was nothing compared to what many people are coping with. In effect. I was living in a bubble: I believed that you could buy fresh food for a similar cost to processed ready-meals. What I had not factored in was the cost of storing the food—people may not have fridges to keep food fresh. Neither had I factored in the cost of cooking the food; you need cooking utensils, pans, cooker and fuel. All of which costs precious money that people do not have. Of course they know that fresh food would be better for them, but they do not have the means to engage in that behaviour.

How then are we to live in line with the 'prevention is better than cure' document, which exhorts us to make the right decisions about the meals we prepare for our families and about creating the right home environments that foster good health? Of course these are 'good things to do', but without change at societal and other levels, these are not choices available to many. As I mentioned earlier, I made judgements about the contents of other people's shopping baskets and the choices those shoppers were making. I now know that for many, these are not choices at all, but were actions driven by the bigger picture, their life context.

So, it seems to me that if the focus of living well is being firmly placed on the shoulders of individuals tasked with self-management, then the likelihood is that they are potentially being set up to fail. If you live in accommodation with no access to cooking facilities, your meal preparation will most likely consist of piercing a plastic top and waiting for a ping to indicate it is cooked. Living well starts 'higher up the stream' to use a phrase borrowed from the NHS long-term plan. Only once we have addressed the bigger issues will individuals really have a choice.

Who Evaluates Self-Management Policy?

Having outlined who writes self-management policy, it is important to consider who evaluates it, for as has been noted by Francis et al. (2018: 12) the self-management approach has been adopted at both strategic and policy levels in a "rapid and largely unchallenged" manner "despite its effectiveness having not been proven". Although Francis et al. (2018) were writing about the New Zealand context, the same comment can be made about the UK; if we struggle to define and measure self-management (as discussed in the last chapter) how then can we be clear about our assessment of its use and value?

In the UK there are two key stakeholders that play an invaluable role in questioning health policy. The Health Foundation and the King's Fund are both charities and they are proactive in calling for change, as well as driving change forward. The King's Fund is an independent charity working to improve health and care in England. Its vision is that the best possible health and care should be available to all. It works towards this goal by undertaking research and analysis with the intention of shaping policy and practice. It also promotes understanding of the healthcare system, for example by translating key government documents into 'lay-friendly' more understandable texts. Likewise, the Health Foundation is an independent charity which aims to ensure that policy development is informed by impartial analysis and evidence. Its mission is to help the UK achieve a healthier population, supported by high-quality health care that can be equitably accessed. The Health Foundation works towards this by giving grants to those working at the front line as well as carrying out its own research and policy analysis.

Both the King's Fund and the Health Foundation have an important role to play in questioning current policy and practice. They work closely with patient stakeholders and encourage exploration of innovative methods to overcome the health challenges facing the UK. It is only through questioning decisions, checking the underpinning evidence base and exploring different options that progress happens. For example, Goodwin and colleagues writing for the King's Fund (2010: 5) questioned the evidence base for self-management. They noted that whilst long-term condition management has become a key priority "relatively little information exists on what constitutes best practice". Similarly, Morgan et al. (2016: 244) based in the UK suggest that it is "not clear how all these promising [self-management] ideas hang together, or whether and how they can be co-achieved".

A third professional body of relevance to the issue of pain self-management is the British Pain Society (BPS). The BPS describes itself on its website as the oldest and largest multidisciplinary professional organisation in the field of pain within the UK. Membership includes doctors, nurses, physiotherapists, scientists, psychologists, occupational therapists and other healthcare professionals actively engaged in the diagnosis and treatment of pain and in pain research for the benefit of patients. The society promotes education, training, research and development in all fields of pain, as well as increasing both professional and public awareness of the prevalence of pain and the facilities that are available for its management. It hosts an annual conference and publishes a quarterly newsletter as well as the highly regarded peer-reviewed *British Journal of Pain*. The society website has a host of useful information for non-members too, both for practitioners and those who are living with pain. At the time of writing the society is leading an awareness and fund raising campaign entitled 'PAIN:LESS' which aims to increase the visibility of pain and to increase funding to find ways to better help those people who live with pain.

So What is Really at the Centre of Self-Management Policy?

Self-management in policy places responsibility firmly on the shoulders of those living with long-term conditions. The original focus of *support for* self-management or *collaboration with* the health profession seems to have been lost. For example, the DHSC document 'Your health, your way' (2009) uses the term 'self-care' (not self-management) and defines it as being about "people taking responsibility for their own health and wellbeing. It includes staying fit and healthy, taking action to prevent illness and accidents, using medicines effectively, treating minor ailments appropriately and seeking professional help when necessary" (p4).

Such a focus runs counter to the approaches recommended by the charities. For example, the King's Fund document authored by Goodwin et al. (2010), 'Managing People with Long-term Conditions', suggests that high-quality care should be a collaboration which involves the use of self-management approaches, in which the clinician's role is not limited to providing support or treatment but includes giving patients the skills and confidence to support themselves and manage their condition (Bachman et al. 2006; Boardman and Walters 2009; Callahan 2001). The aim of such approaches should be to "empower, educate and motivate patients, and not a simple sub-letting of care from the professional to the individual" (Goodwin et al. 2010: 41). Similarly, the Health Foundation (2015: 5) defines self-management support as focusing on ensuring "people receive the full range of support they need to manage the physical, emotional and social impact of their long-term conditions at different stages and ages during their lives". In other words, instead of sole responsibility for self-management being placed on the shoulders of the individual it is seen as a much more collaborative supportive approach.

In stark contrast, the Department of Health (2006) published best practice guidance on self-care. The term 'self-care' was used to encompass both self-care and self-management. Self-care being defined as "individuals taking responsibility for their own health and well-being" and self-management as "whatever we do to make the most of our lives by coping with our difficulties and making the most of what we have". Both of these definitions place all emphasis on the role of the individual, first to take responsibility and second to cope with difficulties. The second definition nods at life-context, but again places all responsibility on the individual to cope with whatever circumstances they find themselves in. Not an easy task for someone on a low income, perhaps reliant on benefits (and the byzantine, judgemental, often inhumane, accompanying system).

Similarly, although the NICE (2012) guideline states that health professionals should get to know the patient as an individual, there is a sting in the tail. Health professionals are also advised to ask the patient how their domestic, social and work situation might impact on their health condition and on *their willingness to engage with health services* (my emphasis). So although there is an attempt to recognise the wider picture, a judgemental approach is still taken with the focus being on the person's 'willingness' to engage. Willingness may have no bearing on this, the patient's life context may mean that they could be very willing to engage, but unable to do so in the way the health professional envisages.

In addition, the NHS (2006) long-term conditions self-care document outlines how self-care will be achieved. To be fair, the report does recognise a need to promote a change in perception about the role of *everyone* involved in supporting people with long-term conditions (Department of

Health 2006: 13). There is also recognition that these changes should not simply focus on the individual and their carer but that change is needed within the health and social care services. However, the focus of the document is on the individual and the report states that the impact of any long-term condition and the individual's ability to optimise self-care is related to six bullet points:

How the individual perceived the severity of their condition compared to how severe it actually is. Implicit in this bullet-point is the judgement that the perception experienced by the person with the long-term condition might not match the 'actual' severity. In the field of chronic pain, according to McCaffery (1968) pain is whatever the person experiencing it says it is. Using the phrase 'compared to how severe it actually is' is insulting and dismissive of the experience of the person who has the pain.

How the condition impacts on the person's ability to live normally. Living normally is not defined. Nor is it always condition-dependent. Normal activities of daily living will likely change each day for each individual living with a long-term condition. A person's ability to 'live normally' will depend on a range of things including how their condition is impacting on them (and this can fluctuate throughout the day), their personal life context, the community in which they live, the systemic challenges they face, as well as how they define living normally. Living in a block of flats where the lift is often out of order will mean that the person with a mobility problem will be less able to carry out their normal daily living because they cannot get outside until the lift is fixed. Although they may find mobility difficult, in this example it is a systemic problem that prevents them from 'willingly engaging'.

The beliefs, understandings, expectations of the condition and the perceived role health services can play in curing, caring or supporting. In this bullet point two issues are merged. The first is focused on individuals beliefs. This is a reasonable focus, there is much in the literature to suggest that our beliefs and expectations can play a role in influencing our health. However it should also be recognised that our beliefs and expectations are in turn influenced by our experiences and life context. Failure to take life context into account could lead to misunderstanding and miscommunication of the reasons behind individual decisions and behaviour(s).

The second issue concerns the perceived role of the health service; the choice of the phrase 'perceived role' has an underlying judgemental tinge to it. Are patients here being accused of expecting too much? Are patients being given mixed messages, for on the one hand there is the message that they expect too much and take more than their fair share and on the other hand, in an earlier document, the Department of Health (2006: 5) report states that patients should be partners in their own care, with the autonomy to "decide what support they need, when they need it and how".

How much the patient participates in or avoids active self-care: Here the agency is clearly placed on the individual. A person who is seen not to participate in active self-care will be deemed non-compliant. This bullet-point places no recognition on the impact of the person's life context. A metric: the amount of participation or indeed, avoidance, is totted up, with no attention paid to underlying explanatory factors to the amount of engagement. The assumption is that it is a person's choice as to whether or not they participate in self-care. The choice, if indeed it is a choice, is frames in binary terms. A patient participates or they 'avoid'. Avoid is an interesting and somewhat 'loaded' term. Avoid suggests untrustworthiness for someone who avoids things is evasive, shirks responsibility, holds back, hides, dodges and so on. This binary reduction to participate versus avoid oversimplifies and firmly places blame on the individual, ignoring systemic, community, economic and other influential factors.

The effect of symptoms, loss of control, loss of role on patients morale, mental health and aspirations: The condition will inevitably have an impact on the person concerned but fails to acknowledge that the extent of the impact might be ameliorated by a more supportive, affluent, life context.

The sixth bullet point is the one that was not focused on the patient. Instead the focus is on "health professionals beliefs and expectations in providing care, cure and support". Whilst undoubtedly important, it also neglects the need for health professionals to look at the patient as a whole, to work collaboratively with the patient and so forth. Patients and health professionals are separated, rather than seen as two essential elements of a collaborative relationship.

Policy then pays lip service to the bigger picture, the life-context, whilst focusing attention on the individual. And the more I read the policies, the less I feel that the patient is at the centre of the policy. Indeed, it seems to me that the key underlying drive behind the push towards self-management is saving money. For example Reidy et al. (2016: 2) note that self-management support "has been declared a priority as an essential element of integrated systems of support for long term conditions and as means of achieving cost-containment". Indeed, in the Department of Health (2006) self-care document, much is made in the introduction of the importance and value of self-care (described as an under-utilised resource) and how the NHS could better support people to self-care. Self-care is important because it helps people with long-term conditions to experience better health and well-being, have better confidence and sense of control. But it is also described as improving medicine compliance, preventing the need for emergency health and social services and preventing unnecessary hospital admissions, with these latter perhaps being the driver for the document development. And whilst I would not quibble with the desire to reduce the need for emergency support and hospital admissions—after all staying well and keeping out of hospital is good for everyone—I cannot help but wonder whether the bottom line is that the policies are designed to be money saving tools. Tools to move patients through the system and then place them firmly outside the system, where they are expected to get on with the job of managing the condition they are living with. I also struggle with the way in which policy has focused on the individual without paying attention to the life context. And remember this is exactly what I did when I began to ponder the apparent ready meal epidemic when I moved to Stoke. It wasn't until I explored the issue further and sought advice from people working in Stoke that I was made aware of a world I had no experience of, yet it was a world that was constraining the options available to the people whose food trolleys I was noticing (and to my shame, judging).

In the same way I made assumptions, I think that the policies do too. In my opinion, it is not possible to separate the patient (the 'self') from the influence of their life context. For someone to live well with a long term condition they will need competence, confidence and support. They will need to have the ability to articulate how they feel, what they are struggling with and what they need. They will need guidance for navigating the welfare system, or to find ongoing affordable, physical rehabilitation. They may need housing that encourages health and well-being. There are many reasons why someone living with a long-term condition may struggle to self-manage, but the policies stubbornly focus attention on the individual at the expense of their life context.

CONCLUSION

It seems to me that the premise underlying self-management policy is that if patients have increased knowledge about how to care for themselves, they will reduce their demand on health services. Patients are presumed to have an "innate capacity for personal agency which outweighs many structural determinants evident in their social contexts" (Francis et al. 2018: 2). In the next chapter we pick up on this assumption, and it is an assumption which I consider to be the reason for the mismatch (gap) between the policy maker expectation and the reality of delivering and receiving self-management programmes.

REFERENCES

Bachman, J., Swenson, S., Reardon, M. E., & Miller, D. (2006). Patient self-management in the primary care treatment of depression. *Administration and Policy in Mental Health, 33*(1), 76–85.

Boardman, J., & Walters, P. (2009). Managing depression in primary care: It's not only what you, it's the way that you do it. *British Journal of General Practice, 59*(559), 76–78.

Callahan, C. M. (2001). Quality improvement research on late life depression in primary care. *Medical Care, 39*(8), 772–784.

Department of Health. (2006). *Supporting people with long term conditions to self-care: A guide to developing local strategies and good practice.* London: Department of Health.

Department of Health & Social Care (DHSC). (2018a). *Prevention is better than cure: Our vision to help you live well for longer.* London: Department of Health and Social Care, Gov.uk.

Department of Health & Social Care (DHSC). (2018b). *Framework agreement between the Department of Health & Social Care and the National Institute for Health and Care Excellence.* London: DHSC, NICE.

Department of Health & Social Care (DHSC). (2019). *The government's 2019–20 accountability framework with NHS England and NHS improvement.* London: DHSC.

Francis, H., Carryer, J., & Wilkinson, J. (2018). Patient expertise: Contested territory in the realm of long-term condition care. *Chronic Illness, 15*(3), 197–209.

Goodwin, N., Curry, N., Naylor, C., Ross, S., & Duldig, W. (2010). *Managing people with long-term conditions.* London: King's Fund.

Health Foundation. (2015). *A practical guide to self-management support: Key components for successful implementation.* London: The Health Foundation.

McCaffery, M. (1968). *Nursing practice theories related to cognition, bodily pain, and man- environment interactions.* Los Angeles: University of California at Los Angeles Students' Store.

Morgan, H. M., Entwistle, V. A., Cribb, A., Christmas, S., Owens, J., Skea, Z. C., & Watt, I. S. (2016). We need to talk about purpose: A critical interpretive synthesis of health and social care professionals' approaches to self-management for people with long-term conditions. *Health Expectations, 20,* 243–259.

Murray, R. (2019). The NHS long-term plan: Five things you need to know. Retrieved   from   https://www.kingsfund.org.uk/blog/2019/01/nhs-long-term-plan

NHS. (2006). *Supporting people with long term conditions to self-care.* London: Department of Health.

NHS. (2019). Long term plan. Retrieved from https://www.longterm-plan.nhs.uk/

NICE. (2012). *Patient experience in adult NHS services: Improving the experience of care for people using adult NHS services.* London: NICE.

Reidy, C., Kennedy, A., Pope, C., Ballinger, C., Vassilev, I., & Rogers, A. (2016). Commissioning self-management support for people with long-term conditions: An exploration of commissioning aspirations and processes. *BMJ Open, 6,* e010853.

CHAPTER 3

Self-Management in Practice: Mind the Gap

Abstract In this chapter I identify and explore the gap between self-management as envisaged in policy, as delivered by health professionals and as received by people living with persistent pain. I explore the barriers preventing health professionals from delivering self-management programmes and those preventing people living with persistent pain from implementing self-management principles. In other words, I explore the policy-practice mismatch.

Keywords Chronic pain • Policy-practice mismatch

INTRODUCTION

Those of us who use the trains in the UK will be familiar with the phrase 'Mind the gap'. It is an electronic announcement made when a train arrives at a platform reminding passengers to take care when stepping across the gap between the train door and the station platform as they step up into or down from the train carriage. In this chapter I identify and explore the gap between self-management as envisaged in policy and as experienced in practice by health professionals and people living with pain. In 2018 Masupe and colleagues wrote an article in which they referred to the House of Care model (Coulter et al. 2013). They wrote:

© The Author(s) 2020
K. Rodham, *Self-Management for Persistent Pain*,
https://doi.org/10.1007/978-3-030-48969-4_3

The concept of self-management in its ideal form should be patient-centred, encompassing the different facets of patient context, multidisciplinary health care teams and a responsive health care system. (Masupe et al. 2018: 41)

The House of Care is certainly a place that we should be aiming for: properly joined up care that takes account of the bigger picture. But as noted in the quote from Masupe and colleagues, this is an ideal. And at the moment, this ideal is far from the current reality. Of course, there is nothing wrong with developing plans that could make things better. There is nothing wrong with setting goals that will be difficult to reach. After all, aiming high is how standards are raised. But standards will only be raised if they are built on a firm foundation, one that is evidence-based and combined with clearly articulated goals. Anyone who has been involved in goal setting knows about 'SMART' goals (see e.g. Bovend'Eerdt et al. 2009), where the 'A' in the acronym refers to the set goals as being achievable. How then is it that self-management policy which health professionals are expected to implement, and people living with chronic conditions are expected to practice, is based in my opinion on two unsound assumptions which make the policy unachievable? The first assumption being that knowledge leads to action, or in other words, if we live with a long-term condition and have increased knowledge about how to care for ourselves, we will reduce the demand we make on health services. The second assumption being that focusing attention on the individual living with a chronic condition without taking into account their life context will result in behaviour change.

Does Knowledge Lead to Action?

At first glance, this seems to be a straightforward question. Of course knowledge leads to action. If we know that doing something is bad for us, then why would we continue doing it? Especially if we are living with something diagnosed as a long-term condition, such as persistent pain. But take a moment to think about your own behaviours. Think about the times when you have tried to change something health-related and failed to do so. Think about how determined you were when you made the decision to make a change. Now think about whether you actually did enact the change, and if you did, how long it lasted for. You had all the information you needed to make a decision to change. You knew it would be better for you to make the change. Yet most of us will not have made a long-term change.

Greaves (2015) reviews qualitative work in the field of smoking and highlights the need to see the bigger picture if we are to explain why people continue to smoke in spite of knowing about the harm it does. She ended the interviews she conducted with women who smoked with this final question: "what would your life have to be like in order for you to not smoke?". The way in which women answered this question gave clear examples of just how much change is required (both internal and external) in order to reclaim a smoke free life. In her review, Greaves (2015) quotes from the work of Jacobson (1986: 93) who interviewed 'Viv'. Viv said:

I can remember when the children were very young, I learned that if I ever sat down, they immediately came and crawled all over me. So to try and have some peace, I used to prop my library book on top of the black fireplace and have my cup of tea and cigarette standing up. That was the only time I felt I'd got some space on my own. That was the real highlight of the day.

Similarly, Tod (2003) asked pregnant women about their smoking experiences and quotes one of her respondents as saying: "To be able to stop, you've got to have a…a bloody good life." This highlights the problem. For these women, it was not simply about stopping smoking. They knew the risks. It was their life context which was affecting their smoking behaviour.

In the following example, we can see how knowledge *did* lead to a change in patient behaviour, but this change was blocked by health professionals who were unwilling to recognise or trust the expertise of the patients concerned. In short, people living with diabetes completed training designed to give them the knowledge and skills to manage their condition. The training had been designed by health professionals and was formally recognised as being an approved training programme. However, Snow and colleagues (2013) concluded that patients who had in-depth knowledge of their condition encountered problems because their expertise was seen as being 'inappropriate'. The researchers concluded that although patient education can give people confidence in their own self-management skills, what it can't do is address the power imbalance between health professional and patient. In their paper they showed what happens when expertise that is taught to patients in one branch of medicine is seen as being non-compliant by those who are not specialists in that field. In other words, well-meaning generalist health professionals blocked access to medication and supplies that the patient knew they needed in order to successfully manage their chronic condition. It is clear then that knowledge alone is not enough to change behaviour, yet much of self-management focuses on education and awareness raising.

CAN FOCUSING ON THE INDIVIDUAL LEAD TO BEHAVIOUR CHANGE?

In health psychology many models have been developed to try to understand or explain how and why people move from poor health behaviours towards behaviours that protect or maintain their health. The most commonly used models are labelled 'social cognitive' in approach. Social cognitive models recognise first that we interpret the information around us, and second that our social context has an effect on our ability to engage in behaviour change. Such models acknowledge that our thoughts and emotions are affected by our immediate social context. In other words, it is the interaction between the social context and the way in which we understand, experience and interpret that context which influences whether or not we engage in behaviour change (Albery and Munafo 2008).

More recently the COM-B model which has been meticulously developed by Michie and colleagues has influenced our thinking about behaviour change. First a taxonomy of behaviour change was developed (Michie and Abraham 2008). This is a really useful tool for it enables the classification of the many different types of approaches to behaviour change interventions. This led to the behaviour change wheel, which itself incorporates the COM-B model and is a tool that is used when designing behaviour change interventions (Michie et al. 2014). As well as being the name of a model, the COM-B is also an acronym which stands for the key elements of the model: 'Capability', 'Opportunity', Motivation' and 'Behaviour'. Without capability, opportunity and motivation it is argued that behaviour change will not be successful. At first glance, this model can seem to be very simple (don't forget though that it has been built on years and years of painstaking research), but it clearly shows that a focus on the individual alone will not result in successful behaviour change. An individual may be capable (informed and have the skills) and motivated, but if they do not have the opportunity (perhaps their life context does not afford them the opportunity), then behaviour change will not be successful.

The problems associated with focusing on the individual are also illustrated by the work of Hinder and Greenhalgh (2012) who observed people living with diabetes as they went about their daily life. They watched how people with diabetes navigated day-to-day diabetes-related issues and then later explored these observations with their participants in conversation. They also took participants to a café or restaurant and invited them to order a meal and a drink. This allowed the researchers to observe how people with diabetes navigated food choice in the 'natural environment' of a restaurant/cafe. Watching participants as they went about their daily life and made choices in the face of challenges highlighted the gaps between diabetes self-management ideals and the everyday practical challenges faced by those living with diabetes. They noticed that the times when their participants did not engage in self-management happened in "contexts where people's material, intellectual or emotional resources were stretched, including poverty, low health literacy, a demanding family or social context or multiple morbidity, and especially where all these factors were present and interacting" (Hinder and Greenhalgh 2012: 13). Common problems included health professionals who did not listen to participants, or who actively discouraged questions, as well as the impact of demands of daily life (childcare, domestic duties, paid employment). The work of Hinder and Greenhalgh (2012) elegantly showed how focusing on the individual alone potentially sets that person up to fail.

Similarly, Finlay and Elander (2016) noted that the UK standard care pain referral pathway has an individualistic treatment focus. The problem with this is that it does not reflect the way in which we tend to cope when we respond to persistent pain. Our coping is undertaken within the framework of wider familial and community-based support structures. Our lived experience of facing our persistent pain is inherently social. Focusing attention on the individual fails to take this into account. Therapeutic interventions delivered in isolation from the life context fail to reflect how we live with pain in our social world (Sullivan 2012). In short, focusing on the individual ignores other key elements of our life context that have impact on how and whether we can engage in self-management practices.

At this point, it is important to highlight that I am not the first to notice this mismatch. The Health Foundation (2011: iv) in its document reviewing the self-management evidence noted that: "When it comes to putting self-management support at the heart of routine healthcare, there is a huge gulf between political rhetoric and the reality of UK clinical practice." Similarly, Kelly and Barker (2016) suggest that in medicine and policy making, discussions about behaviour change are subject to six common errors and that these errors have made the business of health-related behaviour change much more difficult than it needs to be:

1. The assumption that behaviour change is just common sense
2. The assumption that behaviour change is about getting the message across
3. The assumption that knowledge and information drive behaviour
4. The assumption that people act rationally
5. The assumption that people act irrationally
6. The assumption that it is possible to predict accurately.

They provide a clear, articulate and devastating riposte to these six assumptions in their beautifully written paper entitled "Why is changing health-related behaviour so difficult?". Arguably, all of their points fit within my two broad questions: (1) Does knowledge lead to action? (2) And does focusing on the individual lead to behaviour change? In this chapter I build further on the work of the Health Foundation (2011) and Kelly and Barker (2016) and identify three further gaps between policy and practice: (1) differing interpretations of self-management; (2) where is the patient voice? (3) what about those people living with multimorbidity?

Gap 1: Differing Interpretations of Self-Management

As has already been mentioned in both preceding chapters—there is currently no clear definition of what is meant by self-management and because we don't have agreement as to what self-management is, we do not yet have an accurate measure of self-management. How then do we know what self-management looks like? How do we know when someone is self-managing successfully? If there are no clear definitions, then how do we know that when we use the term 'self-management', we mean the same thing as someone else using the same term? This is not easy when you consider that "self-management of chronic illness does not exist in a vacuum, but rather within the context of other people and influences" (Grady and Gough 2014: 27). Indeed, Grady and Gough suggest that self-management represents "an amalgamation of the goals of the patient, family, community and the clinician with everyone working in partnership to best manage the individuals illness, whilst facilitating supportive care" (Grady and Gough 2014: e29). And if goals are to be 'amalgamated' there needs to be a common understanding of said self-management goals. This in turn requires a clear understanding of what self-management is and how it should be implemented. But even more than this—it requires a clear *joint* understanding. If all groups do not share the same understanding, then collaboration will be weak. Indeed, if health professionals and patients have a different understanding of what self-management is, but don't realise that they think differently, miscommunication will occur.

An example of this was provided by Sadler and colleagues (2017) who explored self-management with physiotherapists and stroke survivors, many of whom had been left with long-term health problems. The research team learned that the stroke survivors were unfamiliar with the term 'self-management' but when they were invited to do so, they could provide a definition. Their definition focused on the *practicalities* of doing things for themselves without relying on help from other people. The physiotherapists who were also interviewed were familiar with the term and viewed self-management as a "process in which stroke survivors were expected to take an active role in their rehabilitation and manage their recovery and health" (Sadler et al. 2017: 4). The physiotherapists focused their attention on different elements of self-management: developing patients' technical skills (e.g. walking), knowledge of their condition and goal setting. So the two groups had different ways of understanding the term self-management and this in turn led to a different focus in terms of support offered and sought. Both groups made assumptions about its meaning and their respective roles. It proved difficult for the physiotherapists to support self-management when patient perceptions were so different. In effect, the two groups were wanting the same end result but were not realising that they were taking different routes to get there.

In a recent review of the self-management literature, Russell and colleagues (2018) explored the barriers to, and facilitators of, self-management from the perspectives of Chronic Obstructive Pulmonary Disease (COPD) specialist health professionals and of patients living with COPD. The researchers concluded that patients were ill-informed about their condition, did not know how to recognise and respond to condition-related problems and did not understand illness-related terminology. In contrast practitioners were described as expressing concerns about patients' confidence, literacy and recall, whilst focusing their attention on patient medication. The health professionals also viewed goal setting and the wider self-management context as being outside their realm of competence. Patients reported receiving conflicting information from different health professionals and did not feel they were given the opportunity to ask questions in consultations. They also noticed that medicines were prioritised over lifestyle concerns. In short, health professionals did not feel competent to deliver anything but the traditional biomedical treatment, whilst patients wanted to explore lifestyle issues and gain deeper understanding of their condition, but felt practitioners blocked their approaches. The two groups were essentially talking at crossed-purposes and as a consequence little self-management was being done.

If health professionals are to move out of their traditional role of advice giver and expert and move towards a more collaborative approach, there are consequences, implications and ramifications. Health professionals will need to ask patients about their life context and if you begin to ask how things are for someone, they will expect you to do more than listen, they will expect you to take them seriously and work with them collaboratively to address the barriers they identify. So health professionals need to do more than simply pay attention to the patients' own perspective, interests, values and preferred approaches to directing their lives. They need to learn to work with the patients and to give space for the patient voice.

However, paying attention is not sufficient. Listening to and respecting a patient's choice is important, even though doing so is hard. Indeed, supporting someone to solve their own problems and challenges means allowing them to take responsibility for their own decisions, whilst at the same time ensuring that this person has sufficient information to make an informed choice. Such an approach asks health professionals to move away from their traditional role of expert to that of collaborator. This is not comfortable because the boundaries are less clear. There needs to be give and take and genuine interest in and respect for the others' opinion. At present, this is not happening, for example, Morgan and colleagues (2016) noted that those patients whose preferred approach to managing their condition differed from that of their health professional were more likely to be viewed by the health professionals as being 'difficult' patients.

So if people living with chronic conditions are to be empowered to implement self-management practices, health professionals themselves need to learn a new role. That of collaborator. And herein lies a problem. For example, the Health Foundation (2011) highlighted that many clinicians fail to see why their role should change to support self-management.

Changing roles that have such a strong tradition is not easy. It is not surprising that there is resistance. Practice and policy tend to be about saving money and focusing on managing the condition rather than living well with the condition. If we are to help patients live well with their condition, we need to ensure that we are working with the same understanding of self-management (bearing in mind that this is likely to be different for different patients). Health professionals need to recognise that unlike the example shared by Morgan et al. (2016), a patient choosing to manage their condition in their way is not automatically a 'difficult' patient. In short, we need to give more attention to the patient voice.

GAP 2: WHERE IS THE PATIENT VOICE?

As has been mentioned in Chap. 1, self-management is now considered to be an essential element of support for long-term conditions and as a means of cost containment. In 2016, Reidy and colleagues reported on a study they completed looking at how self-management was understood and made available to patients through local commissioning. They noted that the House of Care model (Coulter et al. 2013) moves away from the traditional medical model towards a more collaborative model, one that takes into account the patient's social and cultural background. There is no doubt that such things are vital to holistic health care. However, the phrase 'takes into account' still has an emphasis on the health professional as expert—as someone who gathers information, rather than as someone who works alongside the person living with the long-term condition, working together to find a way forward.

Let us not be too judgemental though, for collaboration is not easy in our current system. It requires commissioners and health professionals not just to listen to patients, but to hear *and* act on what they are saying. However, what seems to happen is that the patient voice is sought, but only superficially. By way of illustration, Reidy and colleagues (2016) interviewed commissioners and enlisted service users to observe publicly held governing body meetings. Although the public meetings were advertised as having the intention to "put patients at the centre", the reality reported by the service users was far from this. There was no clear and transparent process by which service users could become proactively engaged in decisions made about self-management. Neither was there any signposting to other decision-making meetings that service users could attend and contribute to. So although the stated intention was to include patient/public viewpoints, the way in which the meetings were operationalised blocked the meaningful collaborative contribution of service users. Similarly, during the interviews with commissioners, Reidy and colleagues (2016) noticed that the commissioners were not focusing on their local population needs. Instead, attention was paid to national incentives. They concluded that although self-management was mentioned as a priority, this was little more than lip service. Furthermore, Reidy and colleagues (2016: 9) noted that "contrary to guidance and policy, CCGs [Clinical Commissioning Groups] are not implementing services that have come from the needs of the local population". They continue: "the pressing focus in reality, is on financially driven imperatives meaning that putting self-management support into practice becomes the hurdle at which most commissioners fall" (Reidy et al. 2016: 10). So, our commissioners are not focusing attention on local need, their focus is on national pressures. And worse, they are not listening to service users.

Neglecting to include service users is also something that can be seen in the academic world. For example Effing and colleagues (2016) noted that there was an urgent need for consensus on what defines a chronic obstructive pulmonary disease (COPD) self-management intervention. Seeking agreement on what an intervention focused on self-management should be is commendable. And quite rightly, they convened a panel of 28 international COPD experts. The experts worked really hard together to reach consensus. This is no mean feat, experts by their very nature have strong and clear views about how things should be done—it is how they became experts in the first place. Joining a group to work towards a common aim would have meant putting aside their own agendas and egos and looking at the bigger, more important picture of finding agreement. They would no doubt have shared and contested one another's opinions. The initial definition would have been reviewed and rewritten multiple times until they reached a compromise that they were all willing to agree on. They reached consensus. This is exciting and important. But there were some glaring limitations to the process. To be fair, these are limitations that they openly acknowledged in their paper. First most of the members of the expert consensus group already knew one another—many had published together. Their established relationships, their track record of publishing together might have meant that they developed a form of group think where they were blind to views that differed from their own. Second, there was only one nurse; the remainder of the group consisted of medical practitioners (n = 17), medical researchers (n = 10), physiotherapists (n = 4), psychologists ($n = 3$) and epidemiologists ($n = 8$). As you can see from the figures in the brackets, some of the group ticked more than one occupation. And almost as an afterthought the authors note: "Besides more nurses we will also consider including patients in future processes" (Effing et al. 2016: 53). This to me is disappointing. To seek to find consensus about COPD self-management interventions without including the people who are faced with the task of doing the self-management is a problem. Failing to include the patient voice means that health professionals fail to gain insight into the challenges patients are facing as they try to implement the self-management recommendations. I do not doubt that the group is expert, in both practice and research, but without actually including people who are themselves living with COPD, how can this group claim to have reached consensus about what defines a COPD self-management intervention? How can they be sure that they have captured what it is like to live with COPD? How can they be sure that they know what the challenges are of self-managing when you live with COPD? And how do they know whether the definition they produced is considered appropriate, feasible, manageable, implementable by those whom they expect to put into practice their recommendations?

A third example shows how researchers sought the patient voice, but actually failed to include it because of the method of data collection that was used. The Shaikh and Hapidou (2018) paper starts out really positively with explicit recognition that it is important to find out what patients view as being successful chronic pain treatment. They also highlight the problem that traditionally criteria for patient success is determined and set by health professionals, and that this may not match the outcomes that patients consider to be important. So far so good. But then, as we read on and reach the methodology section we find that the way in which the researchers sought to gather patient views was via a bank of questionnaires. At first glance this may not seem so terrible, but the problem is that the questionnaires were chosen by the researchers and so the focus of the questionnaires reflects the issues that the researchers believe to be important. Scales focused on pain intensity, depression and anxiety, whether patients catastrophised, how disabled their pain made them, whether they were able to reach a level of acceptance about their pain, how they coped and how they felt they had done in the treatment programme.

The only question which could be described as seeking the patients' own viewpoint was an open-ended question: "To what extent have you accomplished your goals?" However, this question assumed that accomplishing goals was something that would be important to the patients. It might not be. And even if it was, what goals are being referred to? Would it have helped to know? Would it have helped to know how the goals were set? Were they decided upon collaboratively? Were the goals focused on life context? Or on managing symptoms? Were they realistic (and in whose eyes)? The authors concluded that they had identified some of the psychological factors "that may be most valued or important to participants in their perceptions of self-improvement" (Shaikh and Hapidou 2018: p155). If I were to play devil's advocate, I would suggest that the findings could be interpreted as showing the values that participants disliked the least from the list chosen by researchers. So although these researchers set out to address a problem in the literature, that of including the patient voice, they did so in a way which only allowed patients to rate things that researchers deemed to be important. Whether the things researchers deemed important were also those things that this group of patients deemed to be important, we still do not know, because their voice was not fully sought and as a consequence, nor was it heard.

The previous examples show instances of research which have inadvertently excluded the patient voice. The following example (which was briefly mentioned earlier in this chapter) shows how the patient voice is sometimes actively discounted. Snow and colleagues (2013) wrote about two diabetes patient education programmes with great acronyms: Dose Adjustment for Normal Eating (DAFNE) and Diabetes Education and Self-Management for Ongoing and Newly Diagnosed (DESMOND). Incidentally, the names DAFNE and DESMOND for me conjure up an image of two sensible, reliable friends who take a reasoned and measured approach to life. I can only assume the choice of names was deliberate! Both programmes have been carefully designed with the intention of helping people living with diabetes to identify their own health risks and then importantly to have the skills to know how to manage them. DAFNE teaches people with diabetes how to adjust their insulin so that they can choose what they eat. Similarly, the DESMOND programme is designed to support the person with diabetes to become an expert in their own self-management. Both programmes are designed to give control to the people with diabetes. It was anticipated that on completion of training that their expertise and their voice would be heard and respected.

The focus is on living well with a condition, rather than managing the condition well. The difference in emphasis here is small, but the implications are large (and discussed at length in excellent papers by Entwistle and colleagues 2018a, b). Living well with something is important and randomised controlled trials for these two programmes have shown improvements in health outcomes for those who have completed them. As a result, the UK National Institute for Health and Clinical Excellence (NICE) recommends that all those with diabetes should have access to this kind of programme. So far so good. What could be wrong with giving people the knowledge, skills, confidence and competence to manage their condition so that they can live well with it?

The problem arises when patients who are educated about their condition because they have successfully completed these nationally recognised and recommended programmes encounter health professionals who are not open to recognising the patient expertise. Such encounters were detailed by the patients who took part in the study conducted by Snow and colleagues (2013). Patients had either completed DAFNE in the past ten years or were about to attend an education course at a DAFNE centre. The researchers used a range of data collection methods including interviews, observation and course participation. The results made for sobering reading. Those patients who had completed the DAFNE training were positive about it and felt better prepared to proactively manage their diabetes. They spoke of the excitement they felt about taking control of their condition. However, their experience post training was disappointing; they mentioned times when their training, knowledge and expertise were actively undermined by health professionals. These patients had been carefully trained. They had completed a nationally approved programme designed to give them a voice and control over their condition. Yet time and again participants in the study gave researchers examples of times when the health profession ignored their expertise, or worse when their expressed needs based on their training were over-ridden.

A common example involved the process of blood testing. Traditionally people living with diabetes test their blood twice a day, but the DAFNE training recommends that they test their blood at least four times a day. This makes sense if they are proactively adjusting their insulin to match their desired diet. The extra information provided by the additional blood tests helps them to better calibrate their insulin and in turn reduces the likelihood that they will have dangerously high or low blood sugars. In addition, when they successfully completed the (NICE recognised *and* recommended) course, all participants were provided with letters to give to their GPs The letters explained why these people need to test their blood more often than would have been traditionally recommended. The letters also explained that since extra blood testing will be conducted there will be a concomitant increase in the patient need for blood test supplies. So this is a *good thing*. The course providers have thought about and pre-empted the likely questions that a GP would want to ask. They have provided patients with a letter that confirms they have completed a recognised and recommended programme and that as a result, they will be completing more blood tests and so will require the GP to prescribe more blood test supplies. Again, so far so good. But what patients were reporting was that their need for extra supplies was often refused, questioned or even ridiculed.

In the paper, a participant 'Julia' spoke about how her GP did not explicitly refuse the prescription, but the GP dispensary halved the amount requested. When Julia queried this she was told that she only needed to do two tests a day. Julia reminded them about the letter from the diabetes specialist and the dispenser responded, "Well I think it's quite ridiculous, you don't need that many" (Snow et al. 2013: 5). The professional was unable or unwilling to recognise a practice that differed from the traditional approach. Even though this alternative approach was recognised and recommended by the UK national body NICE; a national body set up with the express remit to produce evidence-based guidance and advice for health, public health and social care practitioners.

Similarly 'Phil' spoke of how his GP had originally agreed to supply the extra blood test strips but then without warning or explanation took them off the repeat prescription and insisted that Phil came to the surgery every month to justify why he needed so many more blood testing materials than was traditionally recommended. The letter and the fact that Phil had completed a nationally recognised and recommended programme carried no weight. This became a huge problem for Phil; it was not always possible for him to take time off work to come to the surgery. Indeed, nor should it have been necessary to do so. The end result of this obstructive practice meant that Phil felt that he had no choice other than to reduce the number of tests he completed each day, which meant he was unable to monitor his diabetes in the way he had been taught and his blood glucose began to rise again. All because his GP refused to (1) countenance the notion that there was another way of living with and self-managing diabetes, (2) acknowledge Phil's expertise, (3) accept the expertise of the DAFNE diabetes specialist who had written the letter and (4) acknowledge the recommendations from NICE that all people with diabetes should be offered this training.

Another participant Mary said that she no longer went to her GP for diabetes-related issues after an upsetting and, in her view, unnecessary admission to hospital that had been instigated by her GP. She spoke of how her blood sugar reading had been 18 and the GP insisted on calling an ambulance. Mary was not worried because 18 for her was not unusual. But her expertise was ignored. This continued in the hospital where they refused to discharge her. Mary described trying to explain to the hospital staff that because she was "stuck in bed, my blood sugars aren't coming down because I'm stressed, I've got an infection..." (Snow et al. 2013: p6). But stuck she remained. This was such a distressing and undermining experience that Mary now opts to avoid her GP.

So what to make of all this? How can something which on the face of it is positive, has good health outcomes, is even recommended by NICE go so wrong? Snow and colleagues (2013) conclude that until the education of health professionals is considered in parallel with that of patients, these scenarios will continue to occur. They note that although modern health-care practice focuses on patient-centred care, "it does not prepare health-care students for situations in which their patients have more biomedical and practical knowledge than they do about a specific treatment regimen or illness" (Snow et al. 2013: p7). If our health practitioners do not understand a person's self-management requirements and if for whatever reason, they do not trust that person's ability, then they are likely to make self-management unnecessarily more challenging than it already is.

GAP 3: WHAT ABOUT THOSE PEOPLE LIVING WITH MULTI-MORBIDITY?

Kenning and colleagues (2013) paid attention to the important issue of multi-morbidity. They noted that although multi-morbidity is becoming increasingly the norm rather than the exception, the NHS is not generally organised to meet the needs of those with multiple conditions. They wanted to explore how patients and practitioners understood and experienced multi-morbidity with respect to self-management and so they interviewed 20 patients and 20 practitioners. They reported that when practitioners spoke about working with patients with multiple conditions, three key issues were identified: the *complexity* of symptoms and symptom management, the *uncertainty* about how to treat these patients and the *emotional* strain the health professionals experienced when trying to manage patients they labelled as complex and described as showing little improvement or willingness to engage in their own care. As I am writing this section, I have their paper in front of me and I note that I have written the word 'judgy' next to this description. The focus of the health professionals was on their own uncertainty and the stress (emotional strain) they experienced when managing patients with complex health needs. And having practised in the NHS myself I am fully aware of the time constraints health professionals face. But stating that someone is unwilling to engage in their own care is a big label to apply and it is a label that will likely affect how that patient is viewed by other health professionals who read the description in the patient notes.

As an aside, on this specific note of labels, I have recently been completing a short course on cognitive behaviour therapy (CBT) and in the break during one session we were discussing the kinds of patients that might be referred for CBT. Members of the group had heard of patients being referred to services because they were identified as being 'treatment-resistant'. When we sat back thought about this label, we were appalled. The element of blame in that label—that the patients are somehow resistant to treatment—has the subtext that they are actively resisting. The possibility of an alternative explanation, that the treatment they had been offered to date was perhaps not appropriate or practicable for their life context, is ignored.

It was clear that the *practitioners* written about in Kenning and colleagues paper were not working in their comfort zone when working with people with multiple conditions. For patients with single conditions there are often clear protocols and guidelines; none currently exist for people living with multiple conditions. In contrast, *the patients* in Kenning and colleagues study were focused on how their multiple conditions impacted on their physical ability and their emotional response to their condition. They tended to view seeing their health practitioner as something they would do as a last resort and did not go as often as perhaps they would have preferred. How much of this is due to them picking up on the professionals 'judgy' (to use my term) attitude is something which we can only speculate about until further work is done. Nevertheless, Kenning and colleagues (2013) highlighted a large gap between health professional and patient expectations, beliefs and understanding.

People with more than one long-term condition are faced with having to manage multiple medications and self-care activities whilst reconciling information from multiple providers. At the same time, they are monitoring their different symptoms whilst also trying to get on with their lives. Slightam and colleagues (2018) highlight the problems that this causes, not least when treatment plans are being developed. The main issue is that rather than seeing the person first, in their complicated, complex, human entirety, the system is geared up to focus on specific conditions, often in isolation. This means that the daily burdens of managing multiple conditions are generally not taken into account.

Furthermore, the daily burdens that impact most on the person living with their multiple conditions may not be the ones that are focused upon by the health profession. Indeed, there is a mismatch in that patients are of course focusing on the conditions that prove most burdensome for their everyday life, whilst health professionals may focus on what they deem to be the more medically serious condition. These may not be the same thing. Or perhaps the health professionals focus on the condition which their clinic is set up to treat and therefore don't ask about the other conditions that the patient lives with. Our systems have become ever more specialised, and although there are many positives to this, the downside is that it can feel that no one is taking responsibility for overseeing the bigger picture—that everyone is working in their own area, in isolation from the others. And indeed for patients, it can feel like the health professionals are working in isolation from them.

By way of illustration I draw from a paper written by Potter and colleagues (2018). They write of a patient who was fifty-eight years old, living with diabetes, chronic kidney disease and heart problems. She had lived with her diabetes and kidney disease for some time but had recently been diagnosed with heart problems and it was the heart problem with which she was struggling. When she first reported chest pain to her primary doctor, she said she had not been taken seriously. She felt that as a consequence her diagnosis was delayed and her heart muscle further damaged, which in turn reduced treatment opportunities available to her. On top of this, she had also sought support from her doctors to access specialist cardiac care as well as social services (she needed to make her toilet more accessible). She had been denied both sources of support. The advice she had been given by the different health professionals managing her different conditions conflicted. She felt that they were not able to: "consider the impact of her health conditions as a whole; for example she knew that exercise would potentially help her to manage her diabetes but felt unable to do it because of the pain and fatigue caused by her heart disease" (Potter et al. 2018: 139).

Conclusion

In this chapter I have identified the ways in which there is a self-management policy-practice mismatch. Self-management policy and practice both tend to almost exclusively focus on the individual and on symptom management. This is summarised by Paige and colleagues (2016) who note that: "emphasis is placed on the patient's role in treating his or her own disease through symptom monitoring and management, which is often individualised…" (Paige et al. 2016: p22). This focus ignores life context and so makes self-management difficult to implement. For example, Ang (2018: p4) referencing Gallant (2003) notes that "Self-management does not occur solely at the level of the individual—its success is often dependent on influence from family and friends." Similarly, Dwarswaard and colleagues (2015: p202) concluded that "people with a chronic condition are not capable of self-management on their own. Significant others are needed to live a good life with a chronic condition." I go further and suggest that self-management success depends on more than that; the health professionals need to have the same understanding of what self-management means *and* what it is like to self-manage as their patients. Ignoring life context precludes this. Success also depends on the willingness of health professionals to do three things: (1) to recognise that patients have expertise and to value and trust that expertise, (2) to be willing to move away from the traditional model of health professional as expert to a model where health professional and patient combine expertise and work together, collaborate in order to find the best solution for that patient's life context and (3) to shift focus from managing the condition, to managing well with the condition. Without these key ingredients, it is my thesis that self-management can lead to the 'blame, shame and inflame game'. I explore this concept in the next chapter.

References

Albery, I. P., & Munafo, M. (2008). *Key concepts in health psychology*. London: Sage.

Ang, S. (2018). How social participation benefits the chronically ill: Self-management as a mediating pathway. *Journal of Aging and Health*. https://doi.org/10.1177/0898264318761909.

Bovend'Eerdt, T. J., Botell, R. E., & Wade, D. (2009). Writing SMART rehabilitation goals and achieving goal attainment scaling: A practical guide. *Clinical Rehabilitation, 23*, 352–361.

Coulter, A., Roberts, S., & Dixon, A. (2013). *Delivering better services for people with long-term-conditions: Building the house of care*. London: The King's Fund.

Dwarswaard, J., Bakker, E. J. M., van Staa, A., & Boeje, H. (2015). Self-management support from the perspective of patients with a chronic condition: A thematic synthesis of qualitative studies. *Health Expectations, 19*, 194–208.

Effing, T. W., Vercoulen, J. H., Bourbeau, J., Trappenburg, J., Lenferink, A., Cafarella, P., et al. (2016). Definition of a COPD self-management intervention: International Expert Group consensus. *European Respiratory Journal, 48*, 46–54.

Entwistle, V. A., Cribb, A., & Owens, J. (2018a). Why health and social care support for people with long-term conditions should be oriented towards enabling them to live well. *Health Care Analysis, 26*, 48–65.

Entwistle, V. A., Cribb, A., Watt, I. S., Skea, Z. C., Owens, J., Morgan, H. M., & Christmas, S. (2018b). "The more you know, the more you realise it is really challenging to do": Tensions and uncertainties in person-centred support for people with long-term conditions. *Patient Education and Counseling, 101*, 1460–1467.

Finlay, K. A., & Elander, J. (2016). Reflecting the transition from pain management services to chronic pain support group attendance: An interpretative phenomenological analysis. *British Journal of Health Psychology, 21*, 660–676.

Gallant, M. P. (2003). The influence of social support on chronic illness self-management: A review and directions for research. *Health Education and Behaviour, 30*, 170–195.

Grady, P. A., & Gough, R. N. (2014). Self-management: A comprehensive approach to the management of chronic conditions. *Framing Health Matters, 104*(8), e25–e31.

Greaves, L. (2015). The meanings of smoking to women and their implications for cessation. *International Journal of Environmental Research and Public Health, 12*(2), 1449–1465.

Health Foundation. (2011). *Helping people help themselves: A review of the evidence considering whether it is worthwhile to support self-management.* London: The Health Foundation.

Hinder, S., & Greenhalgh, T. (2012). "This does my head in": Ethnographic study of self-management by people with diabetes. *BMC Health Services Research, 12*, 83.

Jacobson, B. (1986). *Beating the Ladykillers: Women and Smoking.* Pluto Press: London, UK.

Kelly, M. P., & Barker, M. (2016). Why is changing health-related behaviour so difficult? *Public Health, 136*, 109–116.

Kenning, C., Fisher, L., Bee, P., Bower, P., & Coventry, P. (2013). Primary care practitioner and patient understanding of the concepts of multimorbidity and self-management: A qualitative study. *SAGE Open Medicine, 1.* https://doi.org/10.1177/2050312113510001.

Masupe, T. K., Ndayi, K., Tsolekile, L., Delobelle, P., & Puoane, T. (2018). Redefining diabetes and the concept of self-management from a patient's perspective: Implications for disease risk-factor management. *Health Education Research, 33*(1), 40–54.

Michie, S., & Abraham, C. (2008). Advancing the science of behaviour change techniques used in interventions. *Health Psychology, 27*(3), 379–387.

Michie, S., Atkins, L., & West, R. (2014). *The behaviour change wheel: A guide to designing interventions.* London: Silverback Publishing.

Morgan, H. M., Entwistle, V. A., Cribb, A., Christmas, S., Owens, J., Skea, Z. C., & Watt, I. S. (2016). We need to talk about purpose: A critical interpretive synthesis of health and social care professionals' approaches to self-management for people with long-term conditions. *Health Expectations, 20,* 243–259.

Paige, S. R., Stellefson, M., & Singh, B. (2016). Patient perspectives on factors associated with enrolment and retention in chronic disease self-management programs: A systematic review. *Patient Intelligence, 8, 21–37.*

Potter, C. M., Kelly, L., Hunter, C., Fitzpatrick, R., & Peters, M. (2018). The context of coping: A qualitative exploration of underlying inequalities that influence health services support for people living with long term conditions. *Sociology of Health & Illness, 40*(1), 130–145.

Reidy, C., Kennedy, A., Pope, C., Ballinger, C., Vassilev, I., & Rogers, A. (2016). Commissioning self-management support for people with long-term conditions: An exploration of commissioning aspirations and processes. *BMJ Open, 6,* e010853.

Russell, S., Ogunbayo, O. J., Newham, J. J., Heslop-Marshall, K., Netts, P., Hanratty, B., Beyer, F., & Kaner, E. (2018). Qualitative systematic review of barriers and facilitators to self-management of chronic pulmonary disease: Views of patients and healthcare professionals. *Primary Care Respiratory Medicine, 2.* https://doi.org/10.1038/s41533-017-0069-2.

Sadler, E., Wolfe, C. D. A., Jones, F., & McKevitt, C. (2017). Exploring stroke survivors' and physiotherapists' views of self-management after stroke: A qualitative study in the UK. *BMJ Open, 7,* e011631.

Shaikh, M., & Hapidou, E. G. (2018). Factors involved in patients' perceptions of self-improvement after chronic pain treatment. *Canadian Journal of Pain, 2*(1), 145–157.

Slightam, C. A., Brandt, K., Jenchura, E. C., Lewis, E. T., Asch, S. M., & Zulman, D. M. (2018). "I had to change so much in my life to live with my new limitations": Multimorbid patients' descriptions of their most bothersome chronic conditions. *Chronic Illness, 14*(1), 13–24.

Snow, R., Humphrey, C., & Sandall, J. (2013). What happens when patients know more than their doctors? Experiences of heath interactions after diabetes patient education: A qualitative patient-led study. *BMJ Open, 3,* e003583.

Sullivan, M. J. L. (2012). The communal coping model of pain catastrophising: Clinical and research implications. *Canadian Psychology, 53*(1), 32–41.

Tod, A. M. (2003). Barriers to smoking cessation in pregnancy: A qualitative study. *British Journal of Community Nursing, 8,* 56–64.

CHAPTER 4

Why Pain Self-Management Might Result in the Blame, Shame and Inflame Game

Abstract This chapter brings to the fore what I see as the (unintended) consequences of the increased focus on self-management in our health service. I explore the patient journey from explaining their pain through to seeking help. I show how important language is in this context and I identify some of what I call the blame inducing barriers to self-management. In short, I highlight how failure to successfully self-manage can lead to blame (ascribed from the health profession to the person living with persistent pain). As a consequence the person living with persistent pain may feel shame and the added (dis)stress that this brings can inflame (lead to a flare up of) their pain experience.

Keywords Blame • Shame • Inflame • Pain-Management • Barriers

INTRODUCTION

The phrase 'self-management' emphasises the self, the individual, the person living with the health condition. In so doing, this places all the responsibility for successful self-management onto the person living with persistent pain. It ignores the context or the background of the person's life, their support network (or lack thereof), their health literacy (or lack thereof), their financial capacity (or lack thereof), their social capital (or lack thereof) and their relationship with their health professionals (or lack thereof). And yet, the person living with pain is expected to cope.

© The Author(s) 2020
K. Rodham, *Self-Management for Persistent Pain*,
https://doi.org/10.1007/978-3-030-48969-4_4

Traditionally, coping is divided into emotion and problem-focused strategies (Lazarus and Folkman 1984). Underpinning both approaches is the notion that the coping processes themselves are neither good nor bad but what is important is that the approach chosen needs to be appropriate for the context. Successful coping then is *context specific*. Indeed, Folkman and Moskowitz (2004) in their overview and critique of the coping literature note that a coping process which works in one stressful situation may fail to help in another because the success is dependent on how far the situation is controllable. And this, the 'controllable-ness' of our situation, of our life context, I think, is at the heart of what I see as a downside of the self-management approach for persistent pain; so much of our lives is beyond our control. The 'bigger picture' things have the biggest impact on what we can or cannot do. We may have a lovely supportive family and friendship network, but if we don't have the financial capital to travel to and pay for facilities that will enhance our ability to self-manage, we are not going to be able to engage with the prescribed self-management programme.

To return to the Folkman and Moskowitz (2004: 758) paper on coping, I thought it was interesting that they pointed out the coping paradox, where even though "most models of coping view the individual as embedded in a social context, the literature on coping is dominated by individualistic approaches that generally give short shrift to social aspects". In other words, although the social context is acknowledged as being influential, the coping literature is just as focused on the individual as the self-management literature. They go on to quote from the work of Dunahoo and colleagues (1998: 137) who described coping approaches as being like the "Lone Ranger, man against the elements" but they also said that even the Lone Ranger had Tonto. So here in the coping literature is an acknowledgement that coping is not something that happens in isolation, nor is it necessarily something that can be done in isolation, yet still we focus our attention in the coping literature on the individual.

Parallels can be identified when you explore the literature focusing in how organisations address mental health issues in the workplace. In his book, *The Work Cure*, Frayne (2019) remembers a poster that was hung in his old workplace kitchen. The poster had a typically uplifting acronym 'GREAT DREAM' to remind anyone who read it to look after their mental health. Each letter was linked to an action that could be taken by whomever read the poster. Frayne writes of the disconnect between the bright and positive styling of the poster which jarred with the tired, dingy, cramped office kitchen. He noted that the sub text of the poster was that concerted organisational and structural change was not required, rather employees should put greater effort into committing to their own self-maintenance and personal well-being. Frayne notes that it is never mentioned that the workplace itself "might create or exacerbate mental health problems; that stress is piped into the environment as efficiently as air conditioning" (Frayne 2019: 30). Instead, as far as our mental health at work is concerned, the onus is on us to take responsibility, and change our behaviour, responses and thoughts, even in the face of things which we cannot hope to overcome without bigger picture change.

This all puts me in mind of a diagram I once saw many years ago when I worked as a lecturer in organisational behaviour. I remember clearly that when I was putting together a session on ergonomics I came across a diagram of how a human should be shaped in order to operate a lathe effectively. Instead of designing the lathe to fit the capabilities of the human, the human was expected to fit the lathe. The shape a human would need to be in order to operate a lathe efficiently was called 'Cranfield Man'. Compared to a 'normal' human, Cranfield Man would need to be: 1.35m tall, have a 2.44m arm span and 0.61m shoulder width. Cranfield Man was written about by Singleton (1964) and if you seek out the paper, you will find a very fine drawing of a squat human with unfeasibly wide shoulders and extraordinarily long arms.

Why, you might wonder, have I remembered this image at this particular point in this book? I think it sums up what it is that people who are expected to self-manage are up against. They are in effect required to take responsibility for coping for something that is bigger than them. For something that they can't reach, or access, or change without influence from policy, from organisations, from government. So just as in the organisational field where people (not organisations) are held accountable for mental health and in the coping world individuals are expected to cope (even though it is known that coping cannot happen in isolation), so too in the pain self-management world, individuals are held accountable for managing their own pain.

Indeed, Osborne et al. (2007: 192), developers of the Health Education Impact Questionnaire, note that "the acute healthcare sector is designed to identify and treat individuals and discharge them back to the community as 'resolved encounters' in a prompt manner". A person living with persistent pain cannot be 'fixed' as is implied by the phrase 'resolved encounter'. Their condition is not resolvable and so in our current system, they are set to fail before they have begun. And so I argue, this is where the blame, shame and inflame game begins.

EXPLAINING PAIN

This 'game' starts with something as basic as trying to explain the level of pain an individual is experiencing. Although there is no objective test for pain and the widely accepted definition of what constitutes pain states that the severity of pain is whatever the person says it is, the International Association for the Study of Pain (IASP) states that pain is always subjective and the British Pain Society on their website states that "only the person in pain can really say how painful something is." Why then do studies exploring differences between patient and professional pain ratings continue to be published? You may well ask why we spend time and effort on this, if the accepted wisdom is that pain is whatever a patient says it is, what is the point in asking a health professional to rate another person's pain? Why can't we simply trust the person in pain?

With this issue in mind, Seers and colleagues (2018: 815) conducted a comprehensive review of the relevant literature and noted that health professionals were often poor at assessing their patients' pain: "patients and clinicians use information largely inaccessible to the other: the patient uses his or her own beliefs about the pain and underlying causes; the clinician uses the patient's behaviour, facial expression and information about the disorder presumed to cause the pain." It is no wonder then that different ratings of pain are identified. Professionals should therefore avoid assuming that their estimated score is accurate—the patient needs to be asked about their own pain. For example, Dow and colleagues (2012: 184) described a 50-year-old woman who had sometimes felt that her doctors did not believe her:

> you're in pain but you are being told by your doctors "No, you haven't got pain, it's just a pain you're feeling in your head". It just destroys you completely and it gives you a double burden to carry and that's what had happened to me and I was destroyed by it

Failure to believe what a patient says results in loss of trust, upset, hurt and emotional damage. Dures and colleagues (2016: 80) quoted participants who said:

I have noticed that when emotional problems are mentioned in the rheumatology department they tend to be ignored, concentrating more on physical wellbeing. (Male, aged 53, lived with arthritis for less than five years)

I don't think those aspects concern the professionals, I've never once in thirty-one and a half years been asked how I am coping. (Female, aged 59 years, lived with arthritis for less than five years)

Similarly, Kool and colleagues (2009) wrote about the difficulty of living with the pain condition fibromyalgia. The invisibility of the symptoms was difficult not just for the person diagnosed, but also for those who interacted with them. In addition doctors were reported as sometimes finding the apparently healthy appearance of the patient disconcerting, whereas friends and family both struggled to understand, whilst at the same time, fiercely defending their loved one from anyone who doubted the veracity of the condition. People with fibromyalgia reported that they felt that medical professionals who did not understand their condition perceived them as 'whiners'. In short, patients found their condition to be stigmatising, not least because they felt that their credibility as a patient was so often questioned.

Even though, as I have already noted, conventional wisdom from pain professional bodies is that pain is whatever the person who is experiencing the pain says it is; over and over again we see that without 'evidence' the person in pain may not be believed. An example from more than 20 years ago illustrates this ability we have to hold two conflicting beliefs at the same time. In 1998, Rochman studied the attitudes of trainee occupational therapists. Trainees were asked to answer true or false in response to pain-related statements. Rochman found that the highest correct score was in response to the statement 'All pain is real'. Eighty-eight percent of trainees agreed with this statement. A similar number (87%) also agreed that "the patient is the best authority on pain sensation". However, around 40% of the trainees also agreed that "visible signs accompany pain and verify it" and that "malingering is common". Such beliefs seem to be mutually exclusive, and yet trainees in this study (and others reference by Rochman 1998) show that it is quite common to hold such mutually conflicting views. The implications of this are worrying for practice.

Judging patients and finding them lacking is (of course) not restricted to the pain field. Granger and colleagues (2009) explored how communication about the management of heart failure was experienced and understood by patients and their physicians. They reported that patients used terms like 'hard work' when describing what was expected of them, whereas physicians felt that patients had not properly engaged even though the instructions they had given them were 'easy'. Patients said it was hard to manage without help, whilst physicians felt that patients did not properly understand their easy instructions and assumed that further repetition of the instructions was necessary. Judgements and assumptions abound and as we will see in the next paragraph from the work of De Ruddere and colleagues, these judgements and assumptions have implications for how patients are treated.

De Ruddere and colleagues have written a series of papers about how people in pain are perceived (e.g. 2011, 2012, 2013, 2014). They have shown that if there is no clear medical evidence to explain a person's pain, others feel less sympathy, are less inclined to help and more likely to downgrade the amount of reported pain. They note that "pain is a social experience" (De Ruddere et al. 2012: 1198). Yet health professionals focus on how the individual manages their pain. Recognition of the social experience is therefore important. In order to explore this phenomenon further, they developed a series of vignettes which they showed to participants. The vignettes either described the presence or absence of medical evidence for the pain reported by the protagonist. First photos were looked at, then videos were viewed. The person featured then had their pain rated by the participant. Some vignettes showed people in obvious pain, others expressed low-level pain.

In a study using these vignettes with participants drawn from the general population (De Ruddere et al. 2013) the findings indicated that people were indeed less inclined to be sympathetic when medical evidence for the pain was absent. Not only that, but the rated inclination to help someone was reduced if there was no medical evidence, even if the protagonist was expressing high intensity pain. This is important because the 'general population' are our friends, our family and our colleagues. They are the people we would turn to if we were experiencing persistent chronic pain. If our pain was persistent and had no 'medical evidence', how confident are we, that our friends, family, colleagues would rally and be sympathetic. Remember too that the 'general population' is also us: me and you. How confident are you that you would rally and be sympathetic to friends, family, colleagues living with persistent pain?

De Ruddere et al. (2014) recognise that the experience of pain is a private experience which is only accessible to the person who is in pain.

This means that trying to understand the private pain experience (which cannot be objectively measured) is difficult for health professionals. They wanted to understand how health professionals reacted to people living with persistent pain and so they recruited 52 general practitioners and 46 physiotherapists. Using a similar vignette approach to that outlined above, the health professional participants were asked to estimate the protagonists pain, how much they thought the person's pain interfered with their daily activities, their own sympathy for the protagonist and their view concerning the likely effectiveness of pain medication. The findings were unequivocal; where medical evidence for the pain was absent, ratings on all measures were lower. The level of pain displayed in the vignette did not influence the ratings, other than to increase suspicion that the protagonists may be exaggerating.

So health professionals also disregard the information given by the person in pain. The notion that pain is whatever a person in pain says it is, is ignored. This also raises concerns for practice and for the patient experience. You would hope that those who act as gatekeepers to further help (GPs) and pain experts (physiotherapists) were not so easily biased. Looking at all of these papers by De Ruddere and colleagues we can see that both the general public and health professionals are influenced by the presence or absence of medical evidence. This is not good news for people who experience persistent pain for whom there is no medical evidence. It gets worse though; in an earlier study completed by the team (De Ruddere et al. 2011), how likeable a person was perceived to be was shown to influence how seriously their pain was taken. Although the team again relied on vignettes (which remove face-to-face cues, interactions and rapport building), they found that patients who were not liked were quite simply not believed. Those who were not liked had their pain estimated to be less intense than those who were liked.

So now it seems that we also have to be likeable in order to convince people of our pain and to be in a good position to access further support? Take a moment and if you do not already live with persistent pain yourself, think about how you behave when you have a headache, or toothache or a hangover or flu or anything that causes pain that lasts for some time. Are you at your best? Are you likeable? Or are you simply seeking a way to lessen the pain you are experiencing. It is not quite the same thing, but Hochschild (1979) coined the term emotional labour to refer to how we manage our emotions and how we are in many situations expected to manage our emotions. One profession specifically referred to in the article was that of flight attendant. No matter how they really feel, they are expected to act in a particular way. All hospitality work involves emotional labour. And it seems, at least in light of the De Ruddere et al. (2011) study, that perhaps we also expect similar efforts from our patients.

To return to De Ruddere and colleagues' likeability study, likeability was manipulated by the descriptions accompanying the vignettes—each vignette was linked to words denoting a positive, neutral or negative personal trait of the protagonist. So a photograph of the 'patient' would be presented, accompanied in this example by positive words, such as 'faithful, honest, friendly'. Although again, somewhat removed from how likeability is assessed in face-to-face interactions, it is not so far from how things might work in clinic. From my experience when notes are passed between clinicians, invariably a quick summary of the patient concerned is offered. It is entirely possible that this handover could influence one's perspective of the patient before you meet them. It is important to explore this further because of the potential impact on treatment offered. We must all become more aware of our own potential bias. Indeed the title of the paper is telling: "When you dislike patients, pain is taken less seriously." Obviously there were limitations to the study—it was completed online, not face-to-face, small numbers and so on. But nonetheless it provides a thought provoking insight into the influence of unconscious bias and how this could impact on the care offered to people living with persistent pain.

The (Perhaps Underrated) Importance of Language

In the previous section, Kool and colleagues (2009) reported that people living with fibromyalgia felt that they were perceived as being 'whiners'. A pejorative term which according to my concise *Oxford Dictionary* means someone who makes petty complaints. Many studies have been conducted exploring how the way we talk about something affects how it is viewed. If we think further afield, the advertising industry has mastered this skill beautifully and estate agents have in the recent past been called into line for their overenthusiastic (exaggerated) claims made when selling property (their Code of Practice for Residential Estate Agents (2011, updated in 2019) makes for interesting reading!). In the pain field, it is common to read about participants in studies who have been deemed to be 'noncompliant'. Other phrases abound: 'patient engagement', 'appropriate decisions', 'good', 'bad' and 'resistant' patients. For example, Koekkoek et al. (2011: 505) note that difficult patients are those that *do not seem* to do their best to get better, they miss appointments, fail to comply "even to the most modest of lifestyle suggestions". Even those who do try hard, but who relapse may be seen as difficult. The authors chose their words carefully, presumably to avoid blaming, but the phrase "even the most modest" is laden with judgement. Who decides what is modest? Modest for whom? If a health professional is stating this is modest, are they properly conversant with the patient's life context? What a health professional may deem as modest, may, for a patient who has social, financial, cultural and environmental constraints, be a gargantuan task.

To further pick up on the importance of language, I turn now to the work of Dariusz Galasinski. He is a Professor of Discourse and Cultural Studies at Wolverhampton University and he has written widely on the impact and importance of language. In a blog piece fizzing with indignation he wrote a response to articles by Chesanow (2015) and Davies (2013) that had been written about 'difficult' or 'challenging' patients. In his blog piece, he points out that patients are often described in the literature as being 'hostile', 'demanding', 'disruptive'. They are thought to have 'unrealistic expectations' and to be "unwilling to take responsibility for their health". Yet health professionals are in Davies' (2013) article described as being 'hungry, angry, late or tired'. In other words, personal factors are accounted for to explain doctors behaviour but not for patients. As Galasinski (2017) puts it "patients are nasty, doctors are overworked" and this state of affairs quite rightly irks him.

I have already mentioned that many of the studies reported by De Ruddere and colleagues have shown that how health professionals view their patients can impact on the way in which patients are subsequently treated. In another example, Sointu (2017) reported on a longitudinal study of American medical students. Sointu was interested in the issue of inequality and explored this through the way in which students described 'good' and 'bad' patients. She found that 'good' patients were seen as actively taking part in their healthcare. They were involved and showed a desire to help themselves get better. But at the same time, they were also expected to let the health professionals help them to get better. In other words, they were compliant and were grateful to receive help. There is clearly room for confusion here—'good' patients should be actively involved, yet passive and grateful. So they are both empowered and disempowered at the same time. In addition to all this:

a good patient is someone that you can talk easily with. Yeah, and just be able to enjoy the visit while doing the things you need to be doing as well. (Sointu 2017: 69)

So in addition to all the work they must put into managing their condition, 'good' patients must also manage the emotions of the health professional and ensure that the encounter is one in which the health professional is made to feel good. 'Bad' patients in contrast abuse the system, are resistant to the doctor's recommendations, don't take their medication or come to follow-up appointments. They are perceived as taking up more time (presumably more time than the doctors feel they are entitled to) and as costing more because they do nothing to help themselves 'get better'. In other words, 'bad' patients make the wrong choices.

Where to begin with this? The language used is stark. 'Bad' patients are patients who 'abuse' the system, are 'resistant' and do the 'wrong' things. But what is not clear is whether the medical students took time to explore the underlying reasons for the 'wrong choices' made. Patients may be labelled as choosing not to come to follow-up appointments, but maybe they were unable to take further time off work, maybe they were unable to access (or pay for) transport to the appointment. Maybe other life events are preventing them from 'complying'. Remember the patient described by Potter and colleagues (2018) in Chap. 3? She was 58, had multiple conditions and tried to exercise in order to manage her diabetes, but struggled because of her heart disease. Would she have been labelled a 'bad' patient by these medical students?

Although some medical students did recognise the influence of resources, or lack thereof, the patients who couldn't follow up because of financial problems were still placed in the 'bad' patient category. Similarly, 'bad' patients were described as poor communicators. For example, they were described as giving one word answers. For example, medical student 'Grace' said:

You ask a question and they kind of stare at you or give you a one word answer, or like seem to have no idea what is going on with their health. (Sointu 2017: 70)

Instead of finding a way to reach the patient, those who struggled to communicate were labelled 'not interested' (Sointu 2017: 71). Intriguingly, 'bad' patients in this study were also those who questioned their doctors. It seems there is a fine line here between saying too little and too much, and that patients need to know how to successfully navigate this. Questioning health professionals could be a sign that a patient is taking an active role in their own care. Questioning a health professional does not necessarily equate to querying the motives or knowledge of the health professional; it may be the way in which the patient is trying to inform themselves to better understand their condition and the reasons for the specifics of self-management recommendations. Perhaps this was a limitation in that the participants were trainees and so potentially felt threatened because of their lack of experience? The difference then between a 'good' and a 'bad' label is dependent on the patients' presentation of self and their ability to manage the emotions of the health professional. Those who attain the label 'good' patient got more time, care and appreciation whilst 'bad' patients were not considered deserving or were assumed to not be interested in taking an active role. In short, the 'good' patients allowed the doctor to act as healer and expert. They also possessed "cultural capital; linguistic facility; proactive attitude toward accumulating knowledge, the ability to understand and use biomedical information and an instrumental approach to disease management" (Shim 2010: 2).

WHAT THEN ARE THE BLAME, SHAME AND INFLAME INDUCING BARRIERS TO SELF-MANAGEMENT?

Let's start with navigating the health service. Anyone who has experience of hill walking knows that even when well prepared with a map and a compass that you know how to use, wet weather gear and emergency supplies, it can feel impossible to find a way through and you can get lost (or 'temporarily navigationally challenged' which is a phrase I was taught when completing my mountain leader training). The same can be said for people living with persistent pain who are likely to find that they have multiple appointments with different specialists. And these appointments are rarely arranged so that they fall on the same day. This means that they need to make repeated visits to the health service—at great cost to them, not just in terms of money, but in terms of time and effort. Often a person who lives with pain finds that their mobility is affected and they no longer drive. This makes them reliant on friends and family for lifts, or they are faced with taking unreliable public transport or using more expensive taxis and so forth. If they are managing to continue to work, multiple appointments mean repeatedly taking time off work, which in turn can cause problems.

Sometimes (sadly, as I write, the more accurate word here would be 'often') simply getting a first appointment with a pain specialist is a challenge; Dow and colleagues (2012: 185) described how a man aged 54 described the high level of frustration he felt at the wait he would have to endure before he could be seen at the pain clinic:

> *And I rang him, the GP up and said, "What's this all about?" and he said "Yes, that's the problem, we've got an eleven month waiting period before you can actually see the pain clinic for your first visit." That seemed quite frustrating and this is one of the better pain clinics in the country that had a lot of resource and here was this waiting period and you think well, why is this happening?*

This is more than frustrating it is plain wrong. We know that the sooner people are taught skills that can help them to function in spite of their pain, the better their long-term outcome. To tell this person that he had to wait almost a year, and in effect put his life on hold, whilst hoping that his pain condition did not worsen or become entrenched while he waited is just not good enough.

Once you are offered an appointment, it is likely to be rushed. Our health system is so squeezed and so as a consequence, our health professionals are also squeezed, which means that even when a patient finally reaches the top of the list and is able to speak to a health professional, they do not necessarily feel any better off. Dures and colleagues (2016: 179) quoted two participants who commented on the rushed nature of consultations:

> *No-one has either the time or the inclination to either answer my questions or have any time to listen to me.* (Female aged 39, lived with arthritis for less than 10 years)

> *I had to cope on my own; I didn't feel I could speak to consultant nurse about my problems as it was always rushed/lacking time and the right questions never asked.* (Female aged 43, lived with arthritis for less than 10 years)

Similarly, Potter and colleagues (2018: 138) highlighted the problems experienced by patients who had had a stroke who wanted to be able to cope, but who were unable to access the support and training they needed:

I was just left then to recover as best I could [...] there's nobody willing to listen and help you with the things that you need the help with. So, you just get on with things as best you can and things you can't do, you have to pay to have done for you.... I had a stroke and again I thought maybe I'd get, at last, get some help, but you don't, it's a waste of time. So I just... I don't bother asking any more, I just let it go.

So patients are trying to access help and then implement recommendations given to them by health professionals but finding it too difficult because they cannot access the support they need. A further example relating to accessibility featured in a news story on the BBC website written by Hamish Mackay (2018) detailing a number of different experiences reported by patients who were expected to self-manage but were, in effect, prevented from doing so. One mother spoke about the time when her four-year old son broke his leg. The child's leg was put in a plaster cast and she and her son were sent home. However, there were no wheelchairs for her to borrow. She said that she asked staff what she should do, but they simply shrugged their shoulders. According to the article, out of 139 NHS wheelchair services, 114 said that they were unable to provide wheelchairs for short-term use. It seems to me that it does not matter how much the mother and her son were willing to engage in a positive and active manner, the lack of resources obstructed any possibility of self-management. Lack of access to appropriate resources trumps such willingness and can lead to the accusation of patients being 'non-compliant'.

In 2001 Campbell and colleagues explored patient non-compliance. They noted that with respect to drug regimens, if patients don't comply there are costs in terms of avoidable morbidity, increased hospital admissions, longer hospital stays, which in turn is a source of frustration for health professionals. The focus of Campbell and colleagues' study was on understanding why it was that some patients did not do their physiotherapy exercises. They found that although participants understood why they *should* do their exercises, many only managed to implement some of the exercises. Those exercises that they did engage with were the ones which they could either more easily embed into their everyday life or were those the patients felt were the most beneficial. This seems eminently reasonable to me. Anyone who has tried to change a behaviour knows how difficult it is to do. Imagine being expected to change your behaviour so you can fit things into your daily routine that perhaps you cannot understand or see any reason for doing so. Perhaps you cannot afford the cost or the time or the travel. Perhaps it just does not fit within the context of the rest of your life. Quite simply, it is not going to happen is it? And indeed, Campbell and colleagues (2001: 137) showed that:

> *non-compliance is usually a reasoned response in relation to a person's perception of their symptoms, their assessment of the effectiveness of the intervention and their willingness and ability to incorporate the treatment into everyday life.*

Campbell and colleagues (2001) called for health professionals and patients to work together to reach shared decisions about recommended treatments. Similar findings were reported by Andrews and colleagues (2015) who focused on the difficulties encountered by people living with persistent pain as they tried to incorporate pacing into their lives. Patient education alone was not helpful. Better collaboration with professionals was called for. This is almost a clarion call to health professionals to question the assumptions they make. Is it that patients are non-compliant or is it that they have made a reasoned decision, based on facts that would be accessible to health professionals if they were able to take the time to ask about them. What a shame then, that almost 20 years on, truly collaborative working is still in its infancy.

So What Can We Make of All This?

Those who live with persistent pain who complete a pain management programme are then expected to have acquired the skills they need to manage, to monitor their symptoms and to play an active role in coping with their pain condition. Indeed, engaging with self-management equates to the health profession assuming that you the patient will take responsibility for managing your condition. Fonte and colleagues (2017) argue that although the process of assuming responsibility is a key self-management skill, the literature has tended to ignore the psychosocial processes that are involved with taking on this responsibility. In their paper, Fonte and colleagues (2017) frame the process of taking responsibility as presenting oneself as an adult. However, in the health context, traditionally patients are expected to show deference to and seek approval from health professionals. Negotiating the health professional-patient relationship whilst maintaining status and autonomy as an adult is not easy—we are conditioned (expected) to become childlike, obedient and deferential when interacting with health professionals. As has been shown by the work of De Ruddere and colleagues as well as Sointu (2017), Snow et al. (2013) and others, interacting as an adult or equal collaborator is not always well-received by health professionals.

Of course it is reasonable to expect people to take some responsibility, but as I have mentioned before, managing, coping with and more importantly living well with a persistent pain condition is not something that can be done alone. Done well, it is a collaborative effort. The focus on self-management in effect ignores the complexity of the problem and over-simplifies it to being something an individual should do. In doing that, this gives space for individual patients to be blamed when they fail to 'comply' with 'easy' instructions and removes the need for health professionals to concern themselves with the life context of their patients. However, I wonder, how can health professionals offer advice, recommendations or instructions unless they have some understanding of the context in which the patient will have to enact them? In the same way that we know behaviour change is not straightforward (even when we know something is not so good for us, we may do it anyway, whether consciously or habitually), why then do proponents of self-management assume that instructions are given and people will implement them? Humans are far from the rational beings we like to think we are.

In short, successful self-management requires so much more than individual behaviour change. And actually, we already know this. In their introduction to a paper on complexity in health services, Greenhalgh and Papoutsi (2018) note that:

> Contemporary healthcare is experiencing several important challenges, including a mismatch between the 'patient in the guideline' and the 'patient in the bed' due to multi-morbidity and interacting sociocultural influences; an inability for 'marginalised' patients to access GP services despite the super-science miracle cures ubiquitous in the media; new staff roles, organisational forms and technologies that sometimes seem to worsen the very problems they were introduced to solve; and the policy sacred cow of integrated care repeatedly proving impossible to deliver in practice. (Greenhalgh and Papoutsi 2018: 1)

The phrase 'sacred cow' refers to something that is immune or above criticism. And indeed, this is what self-management seems to me to have become. Of course the idea is intuitively attractive, but the original idea was *supported* self-management. Somewhere along the line, the 'supported' element has disappeared. As a consequence, when people living

Box 4.1   The blame,
shame and inflame trinity

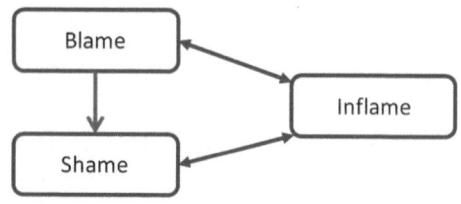

with pain do not implement or incorporate self-management into their daily lives, they are often judged and blamed. They may be described as not compliant, disengaged or difficult. The judgemental attitude which is encouraged by the focus on the 'self' leads to the interconnected trio of 'blame, shame and inflame' (see Box 4.1).

Blame is assigned when the individual fails to implement self-management. Blame may not be explicit, but it is there in the name of the intervention 'self-management'. Failure to embed self-management in your daily life indicates a failure you manage yourself. Shame follows blame. The notion of shame is one which Smith and Osborn (2007) wrote about in the paper exploring how pain impacts on a person's sense of the self. The title of the paper includes the words 'assault on the self' which provides strong insight into their findings. They note that people who feel shame also feel inferior, powerless, that they are somehow less in comparison to other people. Shame has been related to stress in the form of distress and social anxiety (Gilbert 2000). Increased stress is associated with flare ups, where pain is inflamed, aggravated, increased.

CONCLUSION

So what can we do? Smith and Osborn (2007: 529) note that:

> *social and cultural constructs such as culpability, blame and being disbelieved are prominent themes in the experience of chronic benign low back pain, where, in the absence of a clear medical diagnosis of pathology, the sufferer is held responsible for their own condition (Eccleston et al., 1997; Kugelmann, 1997; Osborn & Smith 1998), something Kotarba (1983) referred to as 'victim blaming'.*

This has clear clinical implications. It is important to be supported to move from a state of shame to one of self-respect. Our current system does not yet (in my opinion) consistently and successfully do this. Greenhalgh and Papoutsi's (2018) mention of the 'policy sacred cow' of integrated care being impossible to deliver is both telling and concerning. In the next chapter, I will explore what it is I think we, as individuals and collectively, might be able to do to make things better while at the same time pushing for the systemic, organisational, political and economic changes that also need to happen.

References

Andrews, N. E., Strong, J., Meredith, P. J., Gordon, K., & Bagraith, K. S. (2015). "It's very hard to change yourself": An exploration of overactivity in people with chronic pain using an interpretative phenomenological analysis. *Pain, 156*(7), 1215–1231.

Campbell, R., Evans, M., Tucker, M., Quilty, B., Dieppe, P., & Donovan, J. L. (2001). Why don't patients do their exercises? Understanding non-compliance with physiotherapy in patients with osteoarthritis of the knee. *Journal of Epidemiology and Community Health, 55*, 131–138.

Chesanow, N. (2015). The art of handling 'difficult' patients. *Medscape*, February 23. Retrieved November 25, 2019, from https://www.medscape.com/viewarticle/838283.

Davies, M. (2013). Managing challenging interactions with patients. *BMJ, 347*, f4673. https://doi.org/10.1136/bmj.f4673.

De Ruddere, L., Goubert, L., Prkachin, K. M., Stevens, M. L. A., Van Ryckeghem, D. M. L., & Crombez, G. (2011). When you dislike patients, pain is taken less seriously. *Pain, 152*(10), 2342–2347.

De Ruddere, L., Goubert, L., Stevens, M., Williams, A. C. d. C., & Crombez, G. (2013). Discounting pain in the absence of medical evidence is explained by negative evaluation of the patient. *Pain, 154*(5), 669–676.

De Ruddere, L., Goubert, L., Stevens, M. A. L., Deveugele, M., Craig, K. D., & Crombez, G. (2014). Health care professionals' reactions to patient pain: Impact of knowledge about medical evidence and psychosocial influences. *The Journal of Pain, 15*(3), 262–270.

De Ruddere, L., Goubert, L., Vervoort, T., Prkachin, K. M., & Crombez, G. (2012). We discount the pain of others when pain has no medical explanation. *The Journal of Pain, 13*(12), 1198–1205.

Dow, C. M., Roche, P. A., & Ziebland, S. (2012). Talk of frustration in the narratives of people with chronic pain. *Chronic Illness, 8*(3), 176–191.

Dunahoo, C. L., Hobfoll, S. E., Monnier, J., Hulsizer, M. R., & Johnson, R. (1998). There's more to rugged individualism in coping. Part 1: Even the Lone Ranger had Tonto. *Anxiety, Stress, Coping: An International Journal, 11*(2), 137–165.

Dures, E., Fraser, I., Almeida, C., Peterson, A., Caesley, J., Pollock, J., Ambler, N., Morris, M., & Hewlett, S. (2016). Patients' perspectives on the psychological impact of inflammatory arthritis and meeting the associated support needs: Open-ended responses in a multi-centre survey. *Musculoskeletal Care, 15*, 175–185.

Eccleston, C., Williams, A. C. D. C., & Rogers, W. S. (1997). Patients' and professionals' understandings of the causes of chronic pain: Blame, responsibility and identity protection. *Social Science and Medicine, 45*(5), 699–709.

Folkman, S., & Moskowitz, J. T. (2004). Coping: Pitfalls and promise. *Annual Review of Psychology, 55*, 745–774.

Fonte, D., Lagouanelle-Simeon, M. C., & Apostolidis, T. (2017). "Behave like a responsible adult"—Relation between social identity and psychosocial skills at stake in self-management of a chronic disease. *Self and Identity.* https://doi.org/10.1080/15298868.2017.1371636.

Frayne, D. (2019). *The work cure: Critical essays on work and wellness.* Monmouth: PCCS Books.

Galasinski, D. (2017). Difficult patients. Retrieved November 25, 2019, from http://dariuszgalasinski.com/2017/08/12/difficult-patients/

Gilbert, P. (2000). The relationship of shame, social anxiety and depression: The role of the evaluation of social rank. *Clinical Psychology and Psychotherapy, 7*, 174–189.

Granger, B., Sandelowski, M., Tahshjain, H., Swedberg, K., & Ekman, I. (2009). A qualitative descriptive study of the work of adherence to a chronic heart failure regimen: Patient and physician perspectives. *Journal of Cardiovascular Nursing, 24*(4), 308–315.

Greenhalgh, T., & Papoutsi, C. (2018). Studying complexity in health services research: Desperately seeking an overdue paradigm shift. *BMC Medicine, 16*, 95. https://doi.org/10.1186/s12916-01801089-4.

Hochschild, A. R. (1979). Emotion work, feeling rules, and social structure. *American Journal of Sociology, 85*(3), 551–575.

Koekkoek, B., Hutschemaekers, G., Meijel, B. V., & Shcene, A. (2011). How do patients come to be seen as 'difficult'?: A mixed-methods study in community mental health care. *Social Science and Medicine, 72*, 5040512.

Kool, M., van Middendorp, H., Boeije, H. R., & Geenen, R. (2009). Understanding the lack of understanding: Invalidation from the perspective of the patient with Fibromyalgia. *Arthritis & Rheumatism, 61*(12), 1650–1656.

Kotarba, J. A. (1983). *Chronic pain: Its social dimensions.* London: Sage.

Kugelmann, R. (1997). The psychology and management of pain. *Theory and Psychology, 7,* 43–65.

Lazarus, R. S., & Folkman, S. (1984). *Stress appraisal and coping.* New York: Springer.

Mackay, H. (2018). Wheelchair shortage: "I had to carry my son after he broke his leg". *BBC News Website,* July 27. Retrieved November 18, 2019, from https://www.bbc.co.uk/news/uk-44964130

Osborn, M., & Smith, J. A. (1998). The personal experience of chronic benign lower back pain: An Interpretative phenomenological analysis. *British Journal of Health Psychology, 3,* 65–83.

Osborne, R. H., Elsworth, G. R., & Whitfield, K. (2007). The Health Education Impact Questionnaire (heiQ): An outcomes and evaluation measure for patient education and self-management interventions for people with chronic conditions. *Patient Education and Counselling, 66*(2), 192–201.

Potter, C. M., Kelly, L., Hunter, C., Fitzpatrick, R., & Peters, M. (2018). The context of coping: A qualitative exploration of underlying inequalities that influence health services support for people living with long term conditions. *Sociology of Health & Illness, 40*(1), 130–145.

Rochman, D. L. (1998). Students' knowledge of pain: A survey of four schools. *Occupational Therapy International, 5*(2), 140–154.

Seers, T., Derry, S., Seers, K., & Moore, R. A. (2018). Professionals underestimate patients' pain: A comprehensive review. *Pain, 159*(5), 811–815.

Shim, J. K. (2010). Cultural health capital: A theoretical approach to understanding health care interactions and the dynamics of unequal treatment. *Journal of Health and Social Behaviour, 51*(1), 1–15.

Singleton, W. T. (1964). A preliminary study of a Capstan Lathe. *International Journal of Production Research, 3*(3), 213.

Smith, J. A., & Osborn, M. (2007). Pain as an assault on the self: An interpretative phenomenological analysis of the psychological impact of chronic benign low back pain. *Psychology and Health, 22*(5), 517–534.

Snow, R., Humphrey, C., & Sandall, J. (2013). What happens when patients know more than their doctors? Experiences of heath interactions after diabetes patient education: A qualitative patient-led study. *BMJ Open, 3,* e003583.

Sointu, E. (2017). 'Good' patient/'bad' patient: Clinical learning and the entrenching of inequality. *Sociology of Health and Illness, 39*(1), 63–77.

CHAPTER 5

Re-imagining Self-Management

Abstract In the previous chapters, I have outlined how self-management has come to be viewed as a panacea. I have looked at how self-management is presented in policy, how it is enacted in practice and explored why it could actually have negative consequences for people living with persistent pain. In this chapter, I suggest that our metrics-driven system has squeezed out of the equation the fact that people ('patients') are part of a wider system and that they have their own life context which in turn impacts on their ability to 'self-manage'. I suggest that self-management is a misnomer because no-one can manage their condition alone, and nor should they be expected to do so. Indeed, when self-management was first presented, it was called supported self-management. I then present a series of suggestions exploring how 'self-management' could be 'done' differently within the current limitations of our NHS resources.

Keywords Pain collaborment • Life-context • Pain management

INTRODUCTION

The way our health budget is spent in the UK is described by the National Primary Care Network (2017) who define the population in terms of three categories:

© The Author(s) 2020   73
K. Rodham, *Self-Management for Persistent Pain*,
https://doi.org/10.1007/978-3-030-48969-4_5

- People with multiple conditions and complex needs who comprise 4% of population but consume 50% of healthcare costs
- People with fewer conditions and less complex needs who comprise 18% of the population and consume 35% of healthcare costs
- Mainly healthy people who comprise 78% of the population and consume only 15% of healthcare costs

Taking these figures, 22% of the population need 85% of the budget for healthcare. And this is not really a surprise if you think about it. 78% of the population are 'mainly healthy'. This is a 'good thing'. It is therefore logical to focus our attention on keeping that large proportion of the population healthy whilst also paying attention to increasing or at least maintaining the health of those in the remaining 22%. Of course I am not for one moment suggesting that the 22% could be reduced to zero, but I am suggesting that the number of people falling into the categories where they have most health needs might be reduced if we worked differently. Working differently will require more attention and funding being given to prevention.

Prevention is an important yet neglected part of the puzzle, for example, Marshall (2016), the British Medical Association (2019) and David Buck (2018) writing for The King's Fund set out a clear case that preventive services should be a priority. Right now we devote a very small proportion of our health budget (only 4%) to prevention (Marshall 2016). So why is it that we continue to focus on the wrong end of the continuum? Why are we pushing responsibility onto the individual? And whilst I am mindful that addressing these systemic, economic, cultural, structural, political issues is beyond the scope of this book. I *am* arguing that we would do well to recognise the issues as they are right now and build that into the way in which we work with people who live with persistent pain. I choose to take hope from the clear messages that are beginning to come from professional bodies and charities about what needs to be done. We have in the past made great strides in public health: smoking cessation in public spaces is a case in point. Whilst we need those in power to wake up and think about the policy and budget decisions they are making, we can be lobbying for change.

One thing we can do is to shift our attention away from the individual. A wider lens is needed, although I recognise that it is almost convenient, and definitely commonplace to 'blame' the individual, under the guise of 'helping' them. To return to David Frayne (2019), he provides examples demonstrating how organisations are keen to show they 'care' about their employees by implementing resilience programmes. However, in doing this, employers are in effect stating that their employees are not tough enough to cope; the subtext is that the fault lies with the employee. Employees experiencing stress and ill-health are firmly blamed for not being resilient enough. Running resilience programmes enables the organisation to say they are supporting their employees whilst removing the attention from the organisational processes that may well be causing the stress in the first place. Indeed, focusing on and blaming the individual is not new. By way of example, in a key paper giving an overview of the context to the development of the discipline of health psychology, Michael Murray (2018) writes about the army's response to shell shock in 1916. I am oversimplifying here, but in short, the army was worried about the impact of shell shock on morale and so evacuated the men affected from the front. However, evacuation was a major challenge to maintaining the war effort. As such Murray (2018) quotes MacLeod (2004: 87) who said: "the army command began to favour a psychological model that blamed the individual rather than external factors and by mid-1916, the Army viewed shell-shock as a contagious psychological response of the "weak" to protracted fighting". The condition was reframed and treatment moved from evacuation to temporary respite from battle. Temporary respite consisted of a short rest, followed by returning the men straight to the front line. In this way, blame was laid at the individual soldier's feet for not coping, for being weak and for contaminating others. It was up to the soldier to gather up his courage to go back to the fight or face severe consequences.

On that note, there is a moving memorial at the National Arboretum in Staffordshire to soldiers who were shot at dawn for what at the time was labelled cowardice and desertion but what we now recognise as likely post-traumatic stress disorder brought on by the horrors of what they had witnessed whilst fighting. The UK belatedly pardoned these men and to me the memorial acts as a stark reminder that there are human beings behind the metrics. Indeed, I fear we are in danger of forgetting this. We need to find a way to use the metrics, but not be driven by them. We need to remember there are people behind the numbers and the terminology used. Long-term conditions (pain in particular) tend to have been formulated as something that is costly, burdensome, taking resources away from other areas. In using such language, we risk demonising those with long-term conditions. For example, Barlow and colleagues (2002: 177) summarised the self-management predicament thus (my emphasis):

Longer life expectancy and increasing numbers of people living with chronic conditions accompany the greying of the demographic profile. The burden of meeting the needs of this growing number of people will fall on already over stretched health care services that are struggling to cope with the demands of acute care let alone the needs of those with long term health conditions.

Look at the terminology here. Longer life expectancy (*greying*) is not such a good thing. It is a *burden* on the *over-stretched, struggling* system. The system can't cope with acute care needs *let alone* the needs of those with long-term health conditions. Nearly 20 years ago Barlow and colleagues (2002) were sounding the alarm and issuing their own call to arms. They were bringing to our attention the fact that the way the health care system was (and to a large extent, still is) set up was no longer fit for purpose. It was set up to help those with acute illness, but arguably the greater need now is to help those with long-term, persistent conditions. So how do we continue to provide a service for those with acute needs whilst also meeting the increasing needs of those with chronic conditions? So far, the problem of increasing demands and associated costs of long-term conditions has resulted in a drive to look at how the individual can make changes in their behaviour to self-manage their condition. But what if self-management as we are doing it is not the answer? What if we need to refocus our attention?

WHAT MIGHT REFOCUSING SELF-MANAGEMENT LOOK LIKE?

Entwistle and colleagues (2018a: 48) question whether self-management as it currently operates has too narrow a focus. After all they wonder, if we just look at educating and motivating patients to alter their behaviours so that they are better able to engage in condition control, is this simply reflecting and perpetuating "limited and somewhat instrumental views of patients"? The focus is on managing the condition, not necessarily on living well with the condition. And whilst there is no doubt that behaviour change is, and should be, a core part of learning to live well with a condition and in so doing, reducing the likelihood of it worsening and so, of course, ultimately reducing the cost to the health system, we would do well to remember the huge amount of work led by Susan Michie and colleagues as they have developed, tested and refined the COM-B model.

This model has greatly enhanced our understanding of the influences on behaviour change. Their work has made it very clear that individual capability, opportunity and motivation alone are insufficient to change behaviour. A combination of all three elements at the individual but also the population level is needed (Michie et al. 2014). So what would a refocus look like? Could we move away from self-management with its nominative deterministic focus on the individual, towards something new? Could we move towards 'collaborment'?

COLLABORMENT

Collaborment[1] as I define is a term that combines collaboration and management. A term that has at its core a recognition that an individual cannot possibly manage in a vacuum. A recognition that the patient's life context impacts on their ability to do (or not do) things. A recognition that the person living with the condition has a level of expertise that should be recognised. A recognition that the patient has a nuanced knowledge and understanding of what will work for them in their life context. A recognition that the person living with the condition should be empowered to make informed decisions about how they live their life and manage their condition. Indeed, as patients learn more about their condition and about what works for them, their expertise increases. But, as we noted in the previous chapter, it can be hard for health professionals to accept and acknowledge patient expertise. Indeed, Snow and colleagues (2013: 6) noted that often those patients who have completed an intensive patient education programme (in this case focused on diabetes) have "specific biomedical, experiential and practical knowledge that exceeds that of many health professionals". This should have been something health professionals valued but instead when expert patients tried to self-manage their condition, they experienced serious obstacles from the health professionals who were not comfortable with the patients' high levels of expertise.

What was important about Snow and colleagues' (2013) work was that they explored the reactions of health professionals to formally trained expert patients. These were not patients who had educated themselves

---

[1] After I coined the term I did a Google search and found collaborment as a term exists in the context of cooperative inline gaming http://neoheurism.blogspot.com/

using Google. These patients had completed a formal training programme, recognised by the National Institute for Health and Clinical Excellence (NICE 2011). This professional body even suggests that all people who have diabetes should have access to this kind of structured education (NICE 2011). With this in mind, what the patients in Snow and colleagues (2013: 6) study reported experiencing was disappointing; their self-management attempts were "greatly discouraged or even forbidden by hospital policy". In making sense of this, the authors note that whilst modern health professional training has a focus on patient-centred care, the trainees are not prepared for situations in which the patients have more biomedical and practical knowledge than they do about a specific treatment regime or illness. Similarly, Francis and colleagues (2018) conducted a multiple case study of 16 people with a range of long-term conditions. They also interviewed primary care clinicians. What they found was that patients generally understood the information and advice they received, and indeed worked hard to meet the goals set. But they also spoke of lacking the energy or structural resources to follow through on their commitments. In contrast, from the health professional point of view, it was clear that patients were presumed to have innate capacity for personal agency which would outweigh anything in their social context that could act as a barrier. Furthermore, if a patient made a decision about their behaviour and this decision did not correspond with a physician's advice, that patient was very quickly labelled 'non-compliant'. A really clear example of the problem with being quick to label was given in the paper:

> *Diane could not manage the exercise machines at a hospital pulmonary rehabilitation group due to severe arthritis, so she stopped attending. The feedback letter to her GP labelled her non-compliant without her rationale being sought. Her comorbidities were overlooked, yet she had far more than her asthma to consider when contemplating a self-management programme. She said 'tell me to exercise and I have to take into consideration asthmas, allergies, eyesight and arthritis. Go for a walk—is the footpath even? No tripping and jolting? No things I will not see? Is the wind blowing? Is there space to take a breather? These are not excuses, they are the challenges I face.'* (Francis et al. 2018: 7)

So no one thought to ask how Diane was doing, nor did anyone follow up to find out why she stopped attending. It was easy to label her as 'non-compliant'. Two other patients in the same study reported waiting over 11 months for orthotics designed to help their mobility but both deemed them unwearable when they finally arrived. As a consequence, neither patient wore them, with one saying that she would have "been better off with the bloody shoe box" (Francis et al. 2018: 18). In short, Francis and colleagues (2018) noted that the system seemed to encourage passivity and eventually the patients in their sample gave up trying. Even apparently confident and articulate people felt disempowered. Pushing patients towards passivity, shame and increasing their sense of failure goes against the notion of self-management, and yet, Francis and colleagues (2018: 8) note that:

> the qualities clinicians appeared to value in patients include coping well, listening, not complaining or being difficult, doing their best or making the effort. Taking medicines, making appointment and turning up (whilst not over attending).

In contrast though it is becoming ever more common to have 'expert patients' who are invited to come in and share their experiences with those newly diagnosed. One participant in the study reported by Francis and colleagues (2018) mentioned that she was regularly contacted by health professionals to talk to patient support groups. She said that she loved this role, but that it was very clear to her that her expertise was only valued in the context of talking with patient support groups. When it came to her own health, her expertise was not welcomed and she was forced into playing two roles, that of expert patient for support groups and that of compliant, passive patient for her own health. This was uncomfortable but because of how the system works, she felt forced to switch roles because as far as her own health was concerned, the health professionals would not work in collaborment with her:

> But you try being an expert, sticking up for yourself with these [hospital speciality] guys. They don't like it. They get really shirty. Start treating me like a kid. And they've got the power. I can't tell them to go and get f***ed like I want to do—it might be slightly counterproductive. (Francis et al. 2018: p9)

IS IT POSSIBLE TO TEACH OUR TRAINEES AND OUR EXISTING HEALTH PROFESSIONALS HOW TO WORK WITH PATIENT EXPERTISE RATHER THAN SEEING IT AS A THREAT?

In short, yes! An example comes from Padilha and colleagues (2017) who completed a participatory action-research study. They included 52 nurses and 99 patients living with COPD in Portugal. They noticed that the nurses tended to take a biomedical approach, focusing on the management of the condition. Patients confirmed this when they said things like: "the nurses don't do much to support health-related behaviours" (Padilha et al. 2017: 124). However, after the research team implemented an intervention whereby a researcher was present in clinics in order to stimulate reflection-in-action (thinking about what you are doing, whilst you are doing it), as well as reflection-on-action (retrospective contemplation of what you did, why you did it and how in future you might do it differently), the nurses commented that they had begun to think differently about how they could work with patients collaboratively. What had seemed an insurmountable issue became possible. At the end of the intervention, the nurses' focus moved from one of managing the condition to a model which focused more on self-management skills. In other words, the focus moved from the condition to the patient and how the patient could live well with their condition; one patient said: "Now the nurses respond to my daily life problems. With their help I can do things that I'd already given up doing" (Padilha et al. 2017: p126)

CAN WE REVISE WHAT COUNTS AS A SUCCESSFUL OUTCOME?

In Chap. 1, we saw the plethora of measures used, all focusing on a different aspect of the 'difficult-to-define' 'self-management'. Banerjee and colleagues (2018) identified 14 measures that were used as a proxy measure to assess self-management. Similarly, Packer and colleagues (2018) identified 28 self-management measures. Their results confirmed the findings of others who have lamented lack of consensus on the definition of self-management. Should we continue to seek a measure of the slippery concept of self-management? What it is that drives this search? What would it be like if we accepted that managing well with a condition means different things to different people and that a suitable measure would be one which is patient-centred. Can we accept that there will never be a single measure of a concept so complex, but that we could refine the measures of the different aspects of managing well. In other fields researchers have used the Patient Generated Index (e.g. Martin et al. 2007) to work with what patients consider important. Could these be used in the persistent pain field? In this way, maybe it would not be beyond the realms of possibility that the health professional and the person living with pain could work in collaborment to identify:

- what living well might look like, and
- how the person living with pain would know if they had achieved it.

This is especially important when you consider that studies have shown differences in how patients and health professionals interpret and understand illness. For example, Moore and colleagues (2018) noted that how patients understood their condition influenced their response to it; not just in terms of whether they sought further advice from the health profession, but also whether and how they acted on recommendations for treatment. The researchers also noted that patients who hold an interpretation of illness that is different to that held by health professionals can result in the patients being perceived as 'non-compliant' and 'lazy'. If patients and professionals have differing interpretations of their condition, they will likely have different ideas about what counts as a successful outcome. If health professionals do not try to understand things from the patient's perspective, collaborment will not happen and agreement about what counts as a successful outcome will be impossible.

We know that behaviour change is an essential element of self-management. We also know that behaviour change is not straightforward and yet still we expect patients to self-manage. And at the same time, we fail to empower them to do so, and we do them a disservice by failing to take into account their needs, wants and life context. By way of example, Westland and colleagues (2018) taped and analysed routine primary care consultations between chronically ill patients and nurses. Nurses tended to prioritise the optimisation of patients' medical treatment according to health care standards, they educated patients about monitoring and controlling their condition and gave advice, but they sought little input from patients' own perspective. There was no collaboration in evidence in the consultations.

Similarly, Slightam and colleagues (2018) noted that health professionals were often focused on providing guideline-concordant care whilst patients tend to focus on the aspects of their conditions that were most burdensome or uncomfortable. They found that patients' most burdensome condition was the one that had the most impact on their ability to do the things they wanted. Persistent pain in particular interfered with mobility, employment and activities of daily living. They suggest that health professionals should take the time to find out from the patient what it is like to live with the multiple conditions, to understand the daily burden imposed by the conditions and in turn how this impacts on the priorities of the patient. Quite simply, if a health professional can "address a condition that is causing the patient discomfort, frustration or burden", then in doing so, they could also remove a barrier to that person being able to manage better. After all, what a health professional deems to be a successful outcome may have no meaning for the person living with the condition. Are health professionals really trying to understand things from the patient's perspective? Are they listening *properly*? Are they *hearing* what the patient is saying and do they understand the context in which the patient is living? If not, how can we agree on successful outcomes? How can we move to a focus on living well?

What If We Focused on Enabling People to Live Well with Their Long-Term Conditions?

If we are ever to truly provide patient-centred care, Pickles and colleagues (2018) argue that it is important for our health professionals to think beyond symptoms and treatment. We need to look at the person holistically, to take into account their life context and work in collaborment with them. What might it be like if health professionals looked at the bigger picture instead of focusing on managing the condition. Can we work with our patients to help them manage well, rather than manage the condition well?

Entwistle and colleagues (2018a) argue that there is an important distinction between helping people to manage their health conditions well *and* helping people to live well with their health conditions

Managing health conditions: If the focus is on better management of health conditions, then support is likely to be biomedically framed and narrowly oriented to symptom and disease control. The focus will be on slowing progression, reducing complications and maximising length of life.

Living well: In contrast, when support is understood in terms of helping people to live well with their long-term conditions, disease control is still part of the picture, but a broader perspective is taken which encompasses more flexible aspirations for health and well-being. The focus moves attention to how a person can live well.

Entwistle and colleagues (2018a: 56) argue that if we focus our attention on working with the person to enable them to live well with their long-term conditions, we bring the person who is living with the chronic condition(s) "more fully into view as an active, moral agent, and one whose view of what counts as living well matters". Typically, health professionals focus on managing the health condition whereas patients want to focus on living well. How could we bring these two perspectives closer together? First we need to know what living well means. This is not something that health professionals or governments or policy-makers can determine alone; it requires collaborment. In other words, working with the person who has the task of living well. It also requires recognition that living well will be different for each person. This is an important point to note and was highlighted in the work conducted by Kohut and colleagues (2018) who explored how adolescents living with chronic conditions made use of mentors. The adolescents did not just seek support for managing their illness, but also for everyday life events. Kohut et al. (2018) concluded that the mentors provided hope for the adolescents that they could live the life they wanted *despite having a chronic illness.* This seems to be the main point here—that people living with chronic conditions want to live life well in spite of their condition, rather than being defined by it.

This on the face of it seems self-evident and almost requires a Homer Simpson-esque 'Doh!'. Of course those who live with chronic illness have an understanding of what living well means to them, even if it is different from that prioritised by the health profession. Surely we can see that they are likely to have a better understanding of what might work in the context of their own lives, and how it might work better if they had access to supported self-management? Why then are we not including them in the discussion? This point is made far more articulately by Salmon and colleagues (2011) who developed a method that enabled them to study relationships not just from the perspective of each participant (in this case, the health professional and the patient), but also from the perspective of the researcher who observed the consultation. The reason this was important was that they had noticed that previous researchers had made assumptions about 'good' patient-practitioner relationships. It was known that good relationships were associated with better clinical outcomes. However, it had been assumed that good patient-practitioner relationships were experienced in the same way by both parties. This assumption meant that it had become commonplace for evidence from just one perspective (patient, practitioner or observer) to be used to make inferences about the patient-practitioner relationship as a whole. Furthermore, they also noted that on the few occasions where more than one perspective had been studied, divergences appeared. Why this is surprising is a mystery to me, but since it was a surprise, it is great that this research was completed in order to bring this mismatch to wider attention. Salmon and colleagues (2011) go on to argue in their paper that it is not enough to analyse interactions between patients and practitioners. The perspectives from all of those involved in the interaction also need to be included in order to more fully understand how the interaction is experienced.

LIVING WELL: HEALTH PROFESSIONALS

Moving towards living well requires health professionals to become aware of the potential for unconscious bias to creep into their interactions with people living with pain. In 2004, Kenny explored constructions of chronic pain in doctor-patient relationships. The rationale offered for the study was that "referral to a chronic pain clinic is often the end of the line for many chronic pain patients. Referral usually signals that all medical avenues have been exhausted and that changes in behaviour and attitudes are the primary goals of treatment" (Kenny 2004: 298). In the study patients were simply asked to share their experience of coping with chronic pain, whereas doctors were read a statement:

> We are interested in hearing your views about and your reactions to what we describe as the 'failed chronic pain patient', the patient who has exhausted all medical and psychological avenues of treatment, including attendance at intensive multidisciplinary pain clinics, and whose reported pain and function has either remained unchanged or deteriorated despite intensive intervention, but who continue to seek a cure for their condition. How do you react to these

patients and what do you think are the main issues that need to be addressed in their management?

Well. What a leading question. What a biased question. To me, the subtext is: How dare someone not get better after so much intervention. And how dare that person continue to seek help. When I read this study, I was curious as to why doctors were not simply asked what is your experience of working with patients who are living with chronic pain? Such an open question would allow for all types of experience to be shared. However, not surprisingly, the doctors responses to the leading question were damning (p302): "Oh no, not another chronic pain patient!" and "I'm no longer interested in people who don't get better. As soon as I know what I'm dealing with, I refer on." Patients who had been asked a more open question described terrible encounters. One that stood out for me summed it all up:

> *One specialist I went to, had an egg timer on his desk. As I walked in the door, he turned the time over and said "You have three minutes. Start talking." I had waited three months for that appointment and had sat for one and a half hours in his waiting room.* (p. 301)

Health professionals who hold biased views before they have met with a patient are not going to be capable of listening to or hearing what it is that the patient has to say. The notion of collaborment would not occur to them. In trying to understand where these kinds of responses might originate, I read Hughes (2017) who wrote a short piece about helping patients living with persistent pain and Youngson (2008) who wrote about the impact of subtle differences in focus and how they impact on the way in which health professionals work with patients. Hughes (2017) noted that the typical response to a person with persistent pain is biomedical in nature. In other words, our health professionals are trained to focus on the pathophysiological explanations; once the pathology is treated, the assumption is that the symptoms will be relieved. This is not the case with chronic pain. The symptoms persist. When the biomedical approach does not work, Hughes (2017) suggests that the natural response is to attribute the cause of the pain to the patient's psychology. Similarly, Youngson (2008) in a transcript from his speech given at the Alan Clarke Memorial Lecture argues that it is "doctors who need rehabilitation, not the patients" (2008: p. 10).

Youngson (2008) differentiates between fixing, helping and serving. Fixing is often the only course of action for something acute. Fixing a patient places the doctor as the expert in charge. Patients put themselves into the hands of the health professional in a transactional relationship. Helping is something he describes as seeming laudable, but he cautions us to be aware of the power relationship. A helper is always in a position of power over the person being helped. This is a dependent relationship that takes power away from the patient. Youngson suggests that taking on the role of helper encourages patients to return again and again, because they have no power. Serving on the other hand is a completely different entity. Serving in the sense that Youngson uses it means finding out what is important to the patient and working with them and supporting them to cope with their condition on their terms. He argues that taking this approach in his experience leads to a relationship which becomes one of mutual respect, honesty and openness. Yet whilst Youngson (2008) argues that health professionals could and should learn to serve, Lorig and Holman (2003: 5) note that in many healthcare settings self-management is not seen as a core part of health professional work. They quote a physician saying, "This is not part of our dance"—well, in addition to learning to, to use Youngson's term: 'serve', perhaps it is also time for health professionals to learn to dance to a different tune?

Living Well: People Living with Pain

Carroll and colleagues (2013) set out to explore what coping meant to people living with persistent pain. They noted that in the pain coping literature, coping with pain generally referred to the cognitive and/or behavioural efforts used by people living with pain to manage that pain. However, in their study, the concept of coping had a much more profound and personal meaning for their participants: "pain coping was described as a complex process that could not be isolated from other aspects of life". This is a really important quote for it makes explicit the notion that life context is of paramount importance.

Similarly, Dickson and colleagues (2011) interviewed 17 people with spinal cord injury. The part of their study which is most relevant to this book is the section on post-discharge care. Patients in their study reported being left to "just get on with it". By 'it' they meant their physical, practical and psychological care. Many struggled to cope and reported feeling frustrated at being unable to maintain their fitness post discharge. They spoke of leaving the rehabilitation feeling positive but very quickly began to feel useless and helpless in the face of their deteriorating physical status: "without the necessary resources to sustain it, they seemed beaten by their injuries" (Dickson et al. 2011: p468). I found the same things in a study I completed following up patients who had completed an in-patient pain management programme. They too were initially buoyed up and enthusiastic, but quickly felt isolated and lost confidence on their return home (Rodham et al. 2012). In both studies participants were very clear that this was not a consequence of their lack of motivation but was due to a lack of access to facilities.

Access to facilities can include access to housing. Keene and colleagues (2018) shared the case study of a woman called Regina. Having a secure place to stay meant that Regina could get into a routine. She could set and act on implementation intentions (e.g. I will take my medicine when I get up in the morning). She could only do this because she was no longer moving from place to place. The lack of stable housing had prevented her from being able to self-manage. Once she had stable housing, her ability to self-manage improved. Having a secure base meant that she was no longer having to move from place to place. In turn, this meant that she was able to store her medication on one place. She said:

> That's the first thing I do. I get up, out that bed. It is right there, I already have my medicine, the needles and everything set up.

Around the same time as the work published by Dickson et al. (2011), Dow and colleagues (2012) completed a series of interviews with 46 people who were living with chronic pain.

As well as experiences where patients had not felt they had been taken seriously, heard or listened to, systemic problems such as long waiting lists were a cause of frustration:

> And I rang him, the GP up and said, 'What's this all about?' and he said 'Yes, that's, that's the problem. We've got an eleven-month waiting period before you can actually see the pain clinic for your first visit. (p. 185)

This is, of course, ridiculous. If someone has pain, the sooner they can have guidance about how to cope with the pain in collaborment with health professionals, the sooner they can be engaging in exercises that hopefully will prevent the pain from getting worse.

More recently, Lennox Thompson (2019) studied people identified as living well despite living with persistent pain. They found that their participants had been on a journey to 're-occupy the self' as a means of regaining a sense of self-coherence that the pain had initially taken away. Their participants had first had to make sense of their diagnosis before being able to decide who to deal with it. An active decision to "get on with life as it is now" was important (Lennox Thompson (2019: 5) as was recognising that coping with and living well with pain would be a lifelong process. These findings are similar to those I found when exploring the coping experiences of my patients, many of whom talked about a battle for control, similar to the re-occupying of the self (Rodham et al. 2012) and of putting life first and pain second (Rodham 2015). Lennox Thompson (2019) concludes their paper by noting that clinicians have a key role to play in facilitating patients to live well.

Living Well: The Health System

We know that one in four Americans have one or more long-term conditions (Slightam et al. 2018) and in the UK around 58% of patients going to the GP have multimorbidity. We know that in the UK people with multiple conditions account for 78% of all consultations (Kenning et al. 2013). This means they will need to manage multiple medications *and* self-care activities *and* reconcile information from multiple providers *and* monitor and distinguish between symptoms from their different conditions (Slightam et al. 2018). However, despite multimorbidity becoming the norm, services in the NHS tends not to be organised around the needs of people with multiple conditions but are specialised. Indeed, disease-specific guidelines are plentiful and although aimed at improving care, often contain contradictory advice—what then is someone to do if told to follow the guidelines for each of their conditions? What is a health professional to do if they are encouraging their patient to follow the guidelines (without taking into account the other conditions their patient may be living with)? Our system needs to change.

Conclusion

In my quotations book from the *Oxford Library of Words and Phrases* (1993: 259), I came across the following Tolstoy quote:

I sit on a man's back, choking him and making him carry me, and yet assure myself and others that I am very sorry for him and wish to ease his lot by all possible means—except by getting off his back.

The meaning of the quote is very similar to another quote often attributed to Tolstoy (but for which I cannot find a reference): "Everyone thinks of changing the world, but no-one thinks of changing himself." Both of these quotes capture beautifully how our default seems to be to look externally for answers when we are looking to change things, yet there are things we could do that could begin to make a difference. As a health professional, as policy-makers we tend to do this, we have in the main, looked at what those people living with long-term conditions can do, rather than reviewing what we do and whether what we do is still fit for purpose. We have placed the focus on the individual when what is really needed is collaborment. What might it be like if we could identify how to do things differently? What might it be like if we all took responsibility for addressing the challenges of living well with persistent pain?

References

Banerjee, A., Hendrick, P., Bhattacharjee, P., & Blake, H. (2018). A systematic review of outcome measures utilised to assess self-management in clinical trials in patients with chronic pain. *Patient Education and Counseling, 101*(5), 767–778.

Barlow, J., Wright, C., Sheasby, J., Turner, A., & Hainsworth, J. (2002). Self-management approaches for people with chronic conditions: A review. *Patient Education and Counseling, 48*, 177–187.

British Medical Association. (2019). *Prevention before cure: Prioritising population health*. London: British Medical Association.

Buck, D. (2018). Blog post: Prevention is better than cure, except when it comes to paying for it. Retrieved December 2, 2019, from https://www.kingsfund.org.uk/blog/2018/11/prevention-better-cure-except-when-it-comes-paying-it

Carroll, L. J., Rother, J. P., & Ozegovic, D. (2013). What does coping mean to the worker with pain-related disability. *Disability and Rehabilitation, 35*(14), 1182–1190.

Dickson, A., Ward, R., O'Brien, G., Allen, D., & O'Carroll, R. (2011). Difficulties adjusting to post-discharge life following a spinal cord injury: An interpretative phenomenological analysis. *Psychology, Health and Medicine, 16*(4), 463–474.

Dow, C. M., Roche, P. A., & Ziebland, S. (2012). Talk of frustration in the narratives of people with chronic pain. *Chronic Illness, 8*(3), 176–191.

Entwistle, V. A., Cribb, A., & Owens, J. (2018a). Why health and social care support for people with long-term conditions should be oriented towards enabling them to live well. *Health Care Analysis, 26*, 48–65.

Francis, H., Carryer, J., & Wilkinson, J. (2018). Patient expertise: Contested territory in the realm of long-term condition care. *Chronic Illness, 15*(3), 197–209.

Frayne, D. (2019). *The work cure: Critical essays on work and wellness.* Monmouth: PCCS Books.

Hughes, M. (2017). Strategies for helping chronic pain patients. *BC Psychologists* 6(3)(Summer), 18–20.

Keene, D. E., Guo, M., & Murillo, S. (2018). That wasn't really a place to worry about diabetes: Housing access and diabetes self-management among low income adults. *Social Science and Medicine, 197*, 71–77.

Kenning, C., Fisher, L., Bee, P., Bower, P., & Coventry, P. (2013). Primary care practitioner and patient understanding of the concepts of multimorbidity and self-management: A qualitative study. *SAGE Open Medicine, 1.* https://doi.org/10.1177/2050312113510001.

Kenny, D. T. (2004). Constructions of chronic pain in doctor-patient relationships: Bridging the communication chasm. *Patient Education and Counselling, 52*, 297–305.

Kohut, S. A., Stinson, J., Forgeron, P., Wyk, M. V., Harris, L., & Luca, S. (2018). A qualitative content analysis of peer mentoring video calls in adolescents with chronic illness. *Journal of Health Psychology, 23*(6), 788–789.

Lennox Thompson, B. (2019). Living well with chronic pain: A classical grounded theory. *Disability and Rehabilitation.* https://doi.org/10.1080/0963828 8.2018.1517195.

Lorig, K. R., & Holman, H. R. (2003). Self-management education: History, definition, outcomes and mechanisms. *Annals of Behavioral Medicine, 26*(1), 1–7.

MacLeod, A. D. (2004). Shell shock, Gordon Holmes and the Great War. *Journal of the Royal Society of Medicine, 97*, 86–89.

Marshall, L. (2016). The economic case for preventing ill health. Blog post, July 25. Retrieved December 2, 2019, from https://www.health.org.uk/blogs/the-economic-case-for-preventing-ill-health

Martin, F., Camfield, L., Rodham, K., Kliempt, P., & Ruta, D. (2007). 12 Years' experience with the Patient Generated Index (PGI) of Quality of Life: A graded structured review. *Quality of Life Research, 16*, 705–715.

Michie, S., Atkins, L., & West, R. (2014). *The behaviour change wheel: A guide to designing interventions.* London: Silverback Publishing.

Moore, A. J., Richardson, J. C., Bernard, M., & Sim, J. (2018). Interpreting intra-corporeal landscapes: How patients visualise pathophysiology and utilize medical images in their understanding of chronic musculoskeletal illness. *Disability and Rehabilitation.* https://doi.org/10.1080/09638288.2018.1443162.

Murray, M. (2018). The pre-history of health psychology in the United Kingdom: From natural science and psychoanalysis to social science, social cognition and beyond. *Journal of Health Psychology, 23*(3), 472–491.

National Primary Care Network. (2017). *Improving accountability in the provision of new models of care.* London: National Association of Primary Care.

NICE. (2011). *Diabetes in adults: Quality standard (QS6).* London: National Institute for Health and Clinical Excellence.

Oxford Library of Words and Phrases. (1993). *Volume 1: The concise Oxford dictionary of quotations.* London: BCA.

Packer, T. L., Fracini, A., Audulv, A., Alizadeh, N., Gaal, B. G. I. V., Warner, G., & Kephart, G. (2018). What we know about the purpose, theoretical foundation, scope and dimensionality of existing self-management measurement tools: A scoping review. *Patient Education and Counseling, 101*(4), 579–595.

Padilha, J. M., Sousa, P. A. F., & Pereira, F. M. S. (2017). Nursing clinical practice changes to improve self-management in chronic obstructive pulmonary disease. *International Nursing Review, 65*(1), 122–130.

Pickles, K., Eassey, D., Reddel, H. K., Locock, L., Kirkpatrick, S., & Smith, L. (2018). "This illness diminishes me. What it does it like theft": A qualitative meta-synthesis of people's experiences of living with asthma. *Health Expectations, 21*, 23–40.

Rodham, K. (2015). *Learning to cope with CRPS/RSD: Putting life first and pain second.* London: Singing Dragon.

Rodham, K., Boxell, E., McCabe, C., Cockburn, M., & Waller, E. (2012). Transitioning from a hospital rehabilitation programme to home: Exploring the experiences of people with Complex Regional Pain Syndrome. *Psychology and Health, 27*(10), 1150–1165.

Salmon, P., Mendick, N., & Young, B. (2011). Integrative qualitative communication analysis of consultation and patient and practitioner perspectives: Towards a theory of authentic caring in clinical relationships. *Patient Education and Counseling, 82*, 448–454.

Slightam, C. A., Brandt, K., Jenchura, E. C., Lewis, E. T., Asch, S. M., & Zulman, D. M. (2018). "I had to change so much in my life to live with my new limitations": Multimorbid patients' descriptions of their most bothersome chronic conditions. *Chronic Illness, 14*(1), 13–24.

Snow, R., Humphrey, C., & Sandall, J. (2013). What happens when patients know more than their doctors? Experiences of heath interactions after diabetes patient education: A qualitative patient-led study. *BMJ Open, 3*, e003583.

Westland, H., Schröder, C. D., Wit, J., Frings, J., Trappenburg, J. C. A., & Schuurmans, M. J. (2018). Self-management support in routine primary care by nurses. *British Journal of Health Psychology, 23*, 88–107.

Youngson, R. (2008). Disabled doctoring: How can we rehabilitate the medical profession? *Alan Clarke Memorial Lecture*, November 27, at the Australian and New Zealand Spinal Cord Society Conference, Christchurch New Zealand. Retrieved December 2, 2019, from https://docplayer.net/161017698-Disabled-doctoring-how-can-we-rehabilitate-the-medical-profession.html.

CHAPTER 6

An Invitation to Make a Difference

Abstract In this chapter I set out what I suppose could be the beginnings of 'Pain Collaborment Manifesto' and in so doing, I invite you to think deeply about how and when you might make a change in your own practice. A change that could take us a step closer to a system which helps people in persistent pain to live well rather than expecting them to manage their symptoms. Take a step towards pain collaborment. Put your thinking caps on. Join me.

Keywords Pain collaborment • Manifesto • Invitation to make a difference

INTRODUCTION

Professor Rona Moss-Morris (2013) wrote that coping with a chronic condition was an ongoing process that would never be fully achieved. In saying this, she was recognising and highlighting the fact that chronic conditions by their very nature are rarely static. As such, each person will need to develop, adapt, change and grow their coping strategies in order to deal with each new challenge as it arises. New challenges come in many forms, not all symptom-related. For example, even though the model they developed takes a largely individualist focus, White and colleagues (2018) recognised that successful coping can be influenced by factors outside the control of the individual. These include the condition, the caregiving

© The Author(s) 2020   93
K. Rodham, *Self-Management for Persistent Pain*,
https://doi.org/10.1007/978-3-030-48969-4_6

system, the medical care system as well as social and environmental factors. Similarly, the World Health Organisation (2003) report edited by Richard Wilkinson and Michael Marmot clearly states that social, political and environmental factors influence our general health. And in 2017, Ella Rhodes from The Psychologist reported on a United Nations article which said that "reductive biomedical approaches to treatment that do not adequately address contexts and relationships can no longer be considered compliant with the right to health". Similarly, Eaton and colleagues (2018) noted that the key things which facilitated a person's ability to manage their persistent pain included confidence in their ability, their relationship with the health professional(s), support from their family and friends and access to services. Finally, Peter Kinderman (2019) in his recent book calls for a paradigm shift in how we look at, treat and manage mental health. Whilst his focus is on mental health, what he says is all about seeing the person as a whole and complex being; not as someone reduced to a particular mental health label. As such, what he says is relevant to the point I am making here about our physical health. He notes that:

> If we have problems so serious that we need to be admitted to a secure psychiatric hospital, presumably because there are fears that we might wish to take our own lives, what we need is an environment that gives us hope and optimism, reminds us that we are valued and loved, makes us feel good and is even (perish the thought) a little luxurious and pampered. But instead… we get a shabby cage. (Kinderman 2019: 215)

Kinderman (2019) writes eloquently about the mismatch between what is needed and what is currently available. Similarly, there seems to me to be (a welcome) increase in the numbers of people who are writing about physical health and recognising that we cannot separate the condition from people's life context (see particularly the work of Entwistle et al. 2018a, 2018b; Kristjansdottir et al. 2018; Lennox Thompson 2019). Acknowledging the importance of life context is not rocket science and it is important to point out that none of this is new. We just seem to have lost our way and forgotten what is important. By way of example, in 1887, Pëtr Kropotkin was writing about French and Russian prisons and their failure to prevent crime. He said:

> Healthy municipal dwellings at cost price, education in the family and at school—of the parents as well as the children; the learning by every boy and girl

of a trade; communal and professional co-operation; societies for all sorts of pursuits; and above all, idealism developed in the youths, the longing after what is lifting human nature to higher interests. This will achieve what punishment is absolutely incapable to do.

Replace the notion of prisons and punishment with ill-health, and the message is the same. We need to do what we can to prevent ill-health in the first place. If we are to do that, we need to look beyond the individual. We need to look at their life context. We need to look at where they live, how they live, what their finances are like, whether they have been able to access education, whether they have a job, a profession, a career, whether they have friends and family. And yes, this does sound utopian. But we cannot treat ill health as if it can be separated from this messy thing we call life. If we as a society fail to deal with the bigger picture problems, how is it right to expect individuals to be able to cope regardless of their life context. We need to at least be aware of our patients' social and financial capital. Tim Senior (2018), a GP working in Australia, encapsulated this idea in his recent article:

For 15 minutes I am supposed to chat about control of a disease, and blood tests and medications. The door is closed, and we can talk about tablets and blood tests, keeping the outside world at bay. Eventually though, whatever happened in our consultation, we send the patient back to the environment they came from. For quite a few of our patients, these environments contain the circumstances in which chronic diseases thrive. (Senior 2018)

It seems to me we have compartmentalised and specialised too much. And partly this is reflected in the health systems we have built—we have ever more specialised staff who are knowledgeable about smaller and smaller bits of information. Indeed, I remember watching a BBC documentary series called Island Medics that brought this into stark relief. The doctor who ran the Shetland Island hospital said something along the lines that medical students who came to complete placements at the hospital were at first very much out of their comfort zone when they arrived. This was because unlike hospitals on the mainland which had a series of specialised departments in which students worked, on the island, they needed to be generalists; they needed to be able to deal with whatever health issues the island people presented with. This meant that the trainee doctors had to develop more general skills and be comfortable switching from, for

example, stitching someone's cut head to fixing a broken arm, to perform-
ing surgery. In contrast, on the mainland in the UK, patients are typically
sent to different specialists for each condition they have. No problem
there *if* the separate parts of the system communicate effectively with one
another. But for the most part, they don't.

In the face of all these barriers, it would be easy to say that it is all just
too hard. That the system is too big to change now. That we are just one
small part and that trying to change is futile. At the risk of being clichéd—
we could start with ourselves. What if (to parrot Epictetus) we identified
that things we could change, and changed them? What might those things
be? For example, when I was in practice, our team worked hard to ensure
that patients appointments with different members of the multi-disciplinary
team were all scheduled for one day. Whilst this meant that patients (many
of whom travelled long distances to come to us) had a very long and tiring
day, it also meant that they did not have to make multiple trips to the
hospital. If we had not managed the scheduling in this way, our patients
would have spent a lot of their time travelling to come to appointments
with different health professionals. Spending your time juggling medical
appointments that could be better scheduled is not a good use of any-
body's time.

Whilst we are making those tweaks, alterations and changes, what if we
thought about bigger things for which we could campaign and lobby? An
example in the news as I write is Greta Thunberg. Look at how her one
girl school protest has led to a global movement. Who knows where *our*
changes might lead? We can ALL make a difference. Although I cannot
second guess the things you will identify that you can change, there are
three areas that I think we could focus our attention on: communication,
collaborment and policy.

COMMUNICATION

Communication is a theme that has run throughout this book. It ranges
from listening to one another *and* hearing what it is that we are saying,
through to becoming aware of the impact our choice of words has on
those we are communicating with. For example, Loftus (2011) wrote
about the common usage of the body as machine metaphor in the pain
field. Although the body-as-machine is intuitively easy to grasp, it is not
necessarily a helpful metaphor:

Because many people believe their bodies are just like machines, they come to think that their physical ailments must be fixable, can always be repaired. [...] Such patients can be easily drawn into the downward spiral of searching for a technical fix that they believe must exist and that they must have, going from one health professional to another in a desperate search for a definitive cure. [...]. This is why chronic pain can be so frustrating for health professionals as well as their patients. They are thinking and working with a metaphor that is simply inadequate. (Loftus 2011: 220)

Donovan and Blake (2000) conducted a qualitative study to find out how commonly used words of reassurance were interpreted by patients. In doing so, they overtly recognised that patients and health professionals can have different perspectives following a clinical encounter and that these perspectives were inevitably informed by our own views, beliefs and previous reassurance. What Donovan and Blake (2000) found was that the difference between successful and unsuccessful reassurance hinged upon the patient's perception that the health professional had understood and acknowledged the patient's difficulties. Key to this was the clinician overtly recognising (and showing the patient that they had recognised) the patient's perspective that their difficulties were serious. This is not rocket science, yet we are still not doing well on this—it is not enough to listen and hear, as health professionals we also have to let our patients know that they have been listened to *and* heard.

Similarly, work completed by Barker and colleagues (2009) showed that what were considered common terms by health professionals often had unintended meanings or negative connotations for patients. Many terms were misunderstood or misconstrued. They also found that being familiar with a term is no guarantee that it is understood. Phrases such as 'non-specific back pain' gave lay people the notion that the health professional did not understand the cause of their back pain and did not know how to treat it. Some participants thought that the phrase simply meant that the health professional thought the pain was non-existent. Similarly, the word 'chronic' indicated to many that it meant the condition was very severe. To others it suggested the condition was incurable. Barker and colleagues (2009) concluded that lay participants in their study understood many of the common terms used by health professionals in a different way to that which was meant. Although they were aware of some of the ways in which the patients misunderstood, health professionals often had no idea of the effect some of the words had on lay participants.

In line with the communication theme, time and again studies have reported patients who say they are afraid because their behaviour and their pain have been questioned by health professionals. Yorkston and colleagues (2010) wrote about how patients experienced communicating with health professionals. Their participants spoke of the difficulty they encountered of trying to convey their pain experience when they were very aware that at face value, they looked 'pretty healthy'. They spoke of feeling like they had to convince the health professionals of their pain *and* of its seriousness. They were worried that their reports were not seen as credible by the health professional. These reported fears bring us back to the issue that since there is no clear measure for pain, health professionals should believe the person in front of them when they say they are in pain. However, until we reach this level of acceptance, then Glenton (2003) writing about people living with persistent back pain notes that patients have a difficult line to walk:

> *as long as doctors serve as gatekeepers, not only to healthcare but also directly and indirectly to social acceptance and financial benefits, the back pain sufferer must strive to live up to the doctor's expectations.* (Glenton 2003: 2251)

It is part of human nature to make assumptions about the person with whom we are communicating, but it is also this tendency which can get in the way of clear communication. It can be very hard for us to identify and then suspend our beliefs, so we could turn to Le Vasseur's (2003) call for researchers to become curious. When we become curious we assume that we do not know or understand the issue under study. In taking on this perspective, we become better able to question our prior knowledge and experience. Although written with research in mind, this is relevant for health professionals who are communicating with their patients. Development of a curious attitude would help us step towards finding out about our patient's life context. Le Vasseur (2003: 418) gives an example to show how we might achieve the development of a curious attitude:

> *If, out of our view, someone were to put an object inside a paper bag, the bag might act as a temporary bracket, because it could prevent us from knowing and labelling the object by sight. If we placed our hand into the bag and could not yet recognize the object, we would have a fresh experience of the object without the interference of our prior assumptions and knowledge. Thus, its qualities of roundness or roughness might become more apparent to us. Its contours, tex-*

ture, and temperature would be part of our experience. Let us say that in a few moments, we recognized the object, and our prior knowledge came flooding back into consciousness. 'Oh, it's just a bird's nest!' we might exclaim. However, in the short interval in which we were poised between perception and recognition, we would have possessed fresh experience.

She argues that it is this moment where we are temporarily stripped of our assumptions by our curiosity that a new perception of the object under investigation, or in our case, the patient with whom we are working, might occur. The ability to develop a curious stance towards our patients requires us to engage in reflexive practice. To do this, we need to be able to acknowledge that our own actions and decisions will colour how we see the patient's situation. Failure to take a curious stance could result in us misunderstanding how things are for our patients. This process is not about putting our own preconceptions to one side, rather the focus is on becoming aware of them and their potential influence. Maintaining a curious stance and actively engaging in reflexivity are therefore key skills for practitioners.

The need for a Le Vasseur style of curiosity is beautifully illustrated by the work of Granger and colleagues (2009) who completed a qualitative study of six pairs of adult patients with heart failure and their physicians. In separate interviews both patients and physicians described completing the heart failure regime as work. Both groups reported the same list of tasks and knowledge requirements. But, patients said completing the regime was 'hard work' whilst physicians spoke of patients not participating in self-care even though the instructions they had given them were 'easy'. And whilst in isolation the instructions themselves may well have been easy, embedding them in their life context was what made it 'hard work'. There were more misunderstandings. Patients felt that they understood what was needed in order to complete their self-care tasks, but they also said that they needed help to do so effectively. Physicians on the other hand thought that patients did not understand what the regimen required and assumed that the patients needed more repetition of the knowledge-based instructions.

A final point in this section is made eloquently by Moseley and Butler (2015). They highlight the mixed messages health professionals can give. They give the example of cognitive behavioural therapy (CBT), an approach which is often applied in pain management programmes. Pain management programmes typically have a caveat highlighting that they cannot take the pain away, but they can help people to better cope with their pain. Moseley and Butler (2015) point out the inconsistency in an approach which on the one hand states pain cannot be relieved, whilst also suggesting that through CBT pain can be modified by our thoughts and beliefs. Such contradictions only serve to confuse and highlight the need for health professionals to give a clear and consistent message. They state:

> *we should continue to strive toward understanding this experience of pain, in all its complexity, and that we should explain what we know to those in pain.*
> (Moseley and Butler 2015: 811)

Collaborment

Collaborment is all about working *with* the patient. It is about being prepared to listen to the patient and take seriously their priorities, their wishes and their expertise. Indeed, accepting that patients will often have different priorities to you is an important part of collaborment. Sadly, as has been shown earlier in this book, we have some way to go before we are comfortable accepting that patients might have expertise about their condition. This was exemplified by the work on people who had completed diabetes training and were competent to manage their insulin. Indeed, Snow and colleagues (2013) concluded that patients who had in-depth knowledge of their condition often encountered problems when their expertise was seen as inappropriate in standard healthcare interactions. So although patient education can give people confidence in their own self-management skills, it cannot solve the power imbalance that remains when a health professional (however well-meaning) overrules the patient's stated desire, in the case of diabetes, blocks access to medication and supplies needed by the patient to successfully manage their condition.

This fits well with Helen Salisbury's (2019) think piece 'The Informed Patient' in which she writes about the relationship between patient and doctor in the old-fashioned 'supplicant and defender of wisdom' role taken by the doctor, and how when this role is taken, it results in doctors feeling threatened by patients who ask questions and who have researched things before coming for their consultation. She argues (and I agree) that we should be working towards a relationship which is a meeting between equals who have come together to pool resources in order to solve a problem. Salisbury concludes: "As doctors it is imperative that we find a way to ask: 'What have you found out so far?' Given an opportunity to share, we can together reconcile conflicting explanations of the symptoms." In other words, health professionals could consider the daily burden that conditions impose for patients and become aware of how these issues may affect self-management. They could also remember that for patients clinical outcomes are only one part of living well with a chronic condition (Snow et al. 2013).

King and Hoppe (2013) sum up the situation well. They reported that patients wanted their physicians to explore their ideas about their problem (to listen to them *and* to hear what they were saying). They want their physicians to try to understand them as a whole person and in so doing, to better understand how their problem affects their life (to understand their life context, the unique barriers they face). They want their physicians to tell them what is wrong in plain language (to communicate clearly and in a way that they can understand). They want their physicians to look for common ground and partnership and to agree on the nature of the problem, the priorities and the goals of treatment. They want them to be approachable and share decision-making (they want colloborment). None of these desires are unreasonable, nor are they difficult. Why then are we still not achieving them?

POLICY

This section is one over which it can feel we have little control. But we can exercise our lobbying powers. We could set up or join an existing All Party Parliamentary Group (APPG). At the time of writing (December 2019), there is an All-Party Parliamentary Group on "Health in all Policies". Its purpose is to consider the effects of national public policy on the health of UK populations—particularly on health inequalities between different population groups. Therefore this may be a useful APPG to contribute to in order to bring about change.

Can we rethink how we see our patients? We managed to schedule appointments for the multidisciplinary team on the same day. If we could do it at our hospital, other hospitals could do the same. Can we rethink the length of our GP appointment times? Do we think it is realistic to see, hear and effectively listen to a person in 7–10 minutes? What does this do to the patient? What does this do to the health professional other than cause stress? Is it possible to accept that we will see fewer patients in a day, but that those we do see will have been properly heard and seen. Robin Youngson (2012) wrote a book focusing on this thorny problem called

'Time to Care'. In it he sets out his vision for how we can create time to care, and in so doing he provides examples of where others have succeeded.

Can we reorganise services so they are more suited to multi-morbidity (Kenning et al. 2013)? In the UK, the Royal College of Obstetricians and Gynaecologists has recently (Dec 2019) called for women's services to be located in a 'one-stop-shop' where women can amongst other things; get reliable information about women's health, as well as access to fertility, contraception and abortion services. They also call for an increase in the length of GP appointment times to 15 minutes. Why can we not do the same for people living with persistent pain?

Can we ensure that the notion of collaboration is built into the health professional training programmes and in so doing move away from the traditional 'health-professional-knows-best' approach? This different perspective would go some way towards helping trainees recognise that they can't possibly know everything and that it is OK to work with, and learn from, their patients. For example, Fu et al. (2018) suggest that there is a need to guide health professionals in the art of building partnerships where expectations are acknowledged and tailored information and support are provided. In short, we need to teach health professionals the skills of listening to *and* hearing what is said by our patients.

Can we lobby the overseers of education, those who accredit courses for our health professionals? Can we ensure pain is a core part of the training of all health professionals? For example, Biggs and colleagues (2015) note that pain education is currently a marginal topic and considered a non-essential part of undergraduate medical education. This is not sensible when you consider the figures from the British Pain Society stating that almost half of the population will experience chronic pain. The Advancing the Provision of Pain Education and Learning (APPEAL) task-force therefore recommended the introduction of compulsory pain teaching for all undergraduate medical students. I would go further and suggest that pain management becomes a core part of teaching for *all* health professionals. Similarly, Breivik and colleagues (2013) called for strategic prioritisation and action to improve the knowledge and availability of care for those living with persistent pain. They noted that even though:

> the various attitudinal, educational, legislative, bureaucratic and economic barriers to effective pain management have been well documented by the World Medical Organisation and the World Health Organisation, and others, we believe that at the root of these many problems are a lack of knowledge and

awareness of the huge impact chronic pain has on quality of life of patients and on healthcare resources. (Breivik et al. 2013: 4 of 4)

They suggest there is a need for undergraduate and postgraduate education in pain medicine for all health professionals. They also called for an awareness raising programme for patients and the public focusing on cognitive and educational barriers relating to how to prevent pain, how to self-treat, when to consult a doctor, what to expect and how to access further support. Finally they called for those who make healthcare decisions to be educated about the benefits and importance of multi-disciplinary approaches to helping people live well with pain.

Summary and Invitation

In 2015, the Chronic Pain Policy Coalition published a report detailing how persistent pain affected the population of the UK and crucially included information on local services and access to them. I would argue that we already know what needs to be done, but we feel impotent when faced with the enormity of the task. We know that pain management is something that is best delivered by multi-disciplinary and multi-professional teams (e.g. CSPMS UK 2015). We know that the composition of the teams should be driven by the composition of the needs of the local population. However, as noted in the National Pain Audit (2013) many services fell below national staffing standards and only 40% of the services that had been surveyed in England were sufficiently staffed for multidisciplinary working. Workforce expansion has been recommended time and time again, yet years of underfunding means that our system is in crisis. In addition to lobbying those who have the power to change this, we also need to look closer to home. We need to think about what IS within our power to change, and then change it. With each change, we move incrementally closer to taking the best of the existing self-management approaches, but better embedding them in an approach that sees the whole person and recognises the impact of life context.

Entwistle and colleagues (2018a) note that living well with a condition requires service providers to move away from negative views of people with long-term conditions. By negative, they are referring to seeing such people as needy, deficient and passive recipients of health care. They mean underestimating people's knowledge and aspirations, they mean attitudes and actions that dismiss and undermine people's reasonable efforts to help themselves. They are talking about negative, moralistic judgementalism against patients who do not comply with professionals' advice (remember the woman who was labelled as not engaging whilst health professionals made no attempt to find out why she had dropped out of the service?). Instead they call for a move towards more positive views of people living with long-term conditions. By positive, they are referring to viewing such people as "active partners or asset-bearing co-producers who themselves contribute to the solutions for their health problems" (Entwistle et al. 2018a: 50).

Changing our focus to that of living well with a condition puts the emphasis back on living. It brings the person and what their definition of living well means back to the forefront of care. It takes seriously a person's life context and puts the onus on the health professional to help their patient help them understand this life context. Doing so helps the health professional understand what actually IS available to each individual patient, and no patient will be the same. As Tim Senior (2018: 387) noted:

> *Chronic diseases thrive where there is a lack of money and a lack of power. Of course we must continue to treat our individual patients, but we must also try to improve the circumstances in which people live, to allow them to thrive, rather than their diseases.*

This in turn moves us away from the ugly assumptions we have made in the past, when we have described patients as failing to 'comply' with medical advice. Instead a health professional is more likely to be better informed about the barriers facing their patients in their respective life contexts, and so more able to work with compassion and realistic recommendations. However, until the bigger systemic changes are brought about, there are always smaller steps that we can take, and maybe together these small steps will add up and make a bigger combined difference.

Invitation: Join me—start moving towards collaborment. After all, what is to stop each of us beginning by identifying one thing that we thought we could do that would make a difference, no matter how small? If we each then developed an implementation plan (we know from health psychology that unless we make specific plans it is too easy for us to leave our plans as good intentions and never act on them), and put our thought into practice, we will have made our first change. What if you were to ask yourself right now: "What is one thing that I could change that could make a difference?" What have you identified? Now work out how you can make your change; put a plan together detailing how and when you are going to implement your change. Now do it. Now think of another thing, make a plan for how to implement it and go round that process again. Notice the difference it makes. Share the change with colleagues. Encourage them to do the same. Make a difference.

REFERENCES

Barker, K. L., Reid, M., & Lowe, C. J. M. (2009). Divided by a lack of common knowledge? A qualitative study exploring the use of language by health professionals treating back pain. *BMC Musculoskeletal Disorders, 10*, 123. https://doi.org/10.1186/1471-2474-10-123.

Biggs, E. V., Batelli, V., Gordon, D., Kopf, A., Ribeiro, S., Puig, M. M., & Kress, H. G. (2015). Current pain education with undergraduate medical studies across Europe: Advancing the provision of pain education and learning (APPEAL) Study. *BMJ Open, 5*(8), e006984.

Breivik, H., Eisenberg, E., & O'Brien, T. (2013). The individual and societal burden of chronic pain in Europe: The case for strategic prioritisation and action to improve knowledge and availability of care. *BMC Public Health, 12*, 1229.

CSPMS UK. (2015). *Core standards for pain management in the UK*. London: Faculty of Pain Medicine.

Donovan, J. L., & Blake, D. R. (2000). Qualitative study of interpretation of reassurance among patients attending rheumatology clinics: "Just a touch of arthritis, doctor?". *BMJ, 320*, 541–544.

Eaton, L. H., Langford, D. J., Meins, A. R., Rue, T., Tauben, D. J., & Doorenbos, A. Z. (2018). Use of self-management interventions for chronic pain management: A comparison between rural and non-rural residents. *Pain Management Nursing, 19*(1), 8–13.

Entwistle, V. A., Cribb, A., & Owens, J. (2018a). Why health and social care support for people with long-term conditions should be oriented towards enabling them to live well. *Health Care Analysis, 26*, 48–65.

Entwistle, V. A., Cribb, A., Watt, I. S., Skea, Z. C., Owens, J., Morgan, H. M., & Christmas, S. (2018b). "The more you know, the more you realise it is really challenging to do": Tensions and uncertainties in person-centred support for people with long-term conditions. *Patient Education and Counseling, 101*, 1460–1467.

Fu, Y., Yu, G., McNichol, E., Marczewski, K., & Closs, S. J. (2018). The association between patient-professional partnerships and self-management of chronic back pain: A mixed methods study. *European Journal of Pain, 22*(7), 1229–1244.

Glenton, C. (2003). Chronic back pain sufferers—striving for the sick role. *Social Science and Medicine, 57*, 2243–2252.

Granger, B., Sandelowski, M., Tahshjain, H., Swedberg, K., & Ekman, I. (2009). A qualitative descriptive study of the work of adherence to a chronic heart failure regimen: Patient and physician perspectives. *Journal of Cardiovascular Nursing, 24*(4), 308–315.

Kenning, C., Fisher, L., Bee, P., Bower, P., & Coventry, P. (2013). Primary care practitioner and patient understanding of the concepts of multimorbidity and self-management: A qualitative study. *SAGE Open Medicine, 1*. https://doi.org/10.1177/2050312113510001.

Kinderman, P. (2019). *A manifesto for mental health: Why we need a revolution in mental health care*. Palgrave Macmillan.

King, A., & Hoppe, R. B. (2013). "Best practice" for patient-centred communication: A narrative review. *Journal of Graduate Medical Education, 5*, 385–393. https://doi.org/10.4300/JGME-D-13-00072./.

Kristjansdottir, O. B., Stenberg, U., Mirkovic, J., Krogseth, T., Ljosa, T. M., Stange, K. C., & Ruland, C. M. (2018). Personal strengths reported by people with chronic illness: A qualitative study. *Health Expectations, 21*(4), 787–795.

Le Vasseur, J. J. (2003). The problem of bracketing in phenomenology. *Qualitative Health Research, 13*, 408–420.

Lennox Thompson, B. (2019). Living well with chronic pain: A classical grounded theory. *Disability and Rehabilitation*. https://doi.org/10.1080/0963828 8.2018.1517195.

Loftus, S. (2011). Pain and its metaphors: A dialogical approach. *Journal of Medical Humanities, 31*, 213–230.

Moseley, G. L., & Butler, D. S. (2015). Fifteen years of explaining pain: The past, present and future. *The Journal of Pain, 16*(9), 807–813.

Moss-Morris, R. (2013). Adjusting to chronic illness: Time for a unified theory. *British Journal of Health Psychology, 18*, 681–686.

National Pain Audit. (2013). *National Pain Audit Final Report, 2010–2012*. London: The British Pain Society.

Salisbury, H. (2019). Helen Salisbury: The informed patient. *BMJ, 364*, l638.

Senior, T. (2018). How chronic diseases thrive. *British Journal of General Practice*. https://doi.org/10.3399/bjgp18X698237.

Snow, R., Humphrey, C., & Sandall, J. (2013). What happens when patients know more than their doctors? Experiences of heath interactions after diabetes patient education: A qualitative patient-led study. *BMJ Open, 3*, e003583.

White, K., Issac, M. S. M., Kamoun, C., Leygues, J., & Cohn, S. (2018). The THRIVE model: A framework and review of internal and external predictors of coping with chronic illness. *Health Psychology Open*, Jul-Dec, 1–14. https://doi.org/10.1177/2055102918793552.

Wilkinson, R., & Marmot, M. (Eds.). (2003). *Social determinants of health: The solid facts.* World Health Organisation.

Yorkston, K. M., Johnson, K., Boesflug, E., Skala, J., & Amtmann, D. (2010). Communicating about the experience of pain and fatigue in disability. *Quality of Life Research, 19,* 243–251.

Youngson, R. (2012). *Time to care: How to love your patients and your job.* New Zealand: Rebelheart Publishers.

REFERENCES

Albery, I. P., & Munafo, M. (2008). *Key concepts in health psychology*. London: Sage.

Andrews, N. E., Strong, J., Meredith, P. J., Gordon, K., & Bagraith, K. S. (2015). "It's very hard to change yourself": An exploration of overactivity in people with chronic pain using an interpretative phenomenological analysis. *Pain, 156*(7), 1215–1231.

Ang, S. (2018). How social participation benefits the chronically ill: Self-management as a mediating pathway. *Journal of Aging and Health*. https://doi.org/10.1177/0898264318761909.

Bachman, J., Swenson, S., Reardon, M. E., & Miller, D. (2006). Patient self-management in the primary care treatment of depression. *Administration and Policy in Mental Health, 33*(1), 76–85.

Banerjee, A., Hendrick, P., Bhattacharjee, P., & Blake, H. (2018). A systematic review of outcome measures utilised to assess self-management in clinical trials in patients with chronic pain. *Patient Education and Counseling, 101*(5), 767–778.

Barker, K. L., Reid, M., & Lowe, C. J. M. (2009). Divided by a lack of common knowledge? A qualitative study exploring the use of language by health professionals treating back pain. *BMC Musculoskeletal Disorders, 10*, 123. https://doi.org/10.1186/1471-2474-10-123.

Barlow, J., Wright, C., Sheasby, J., Turner, A., & Hainsworth, J. (2002). Self-management approaches for people with chronic conditions: A review. *Patient Education and Counseling, 48*, 177–187.

Berne, E. (1964). *Games people play*. New York: Grove Press.

Bernhofer, E. (2011, October 25). Ethics: Ethics and pain management in hospitalized patients. *The Online Journal of Issues in Nursing, 17*(1), 11.

Biggs, E. V., Batelli, V., Gordon, D., Kopf, A., Ribeiro, S., Puig, M. M., & Kress, H. G. (2015). Current pain education with undergraduate medical studies across Europe: Advancing the provision of pain education and learning (APPEAL) Study. *BMJ Open, 5*(8), e006984.

Boardman, J., & Walters, P. (2009). Managing depression in primary care: It's not only what you, it's the way that you do it. *British Journal of General Practice, 59*(559), 76–78.

Borg, K. (2018). Narrating disability, trauma and pain: The doing and undoing of self in language. *A Journal of Literary Studies and Linguistics, VIII,* 169–186.

Bovend'Eerdt, T. J., Botell, R. E., & Wade, D. (2009). Writing SMART rehabilitation goals and achieving goal attainment scaling: A practical guide. *Clinical Rehabilitation, 23,* 352–361.

Breivik, H., Eisenberg, E., & O'Brien, T. (2013). The individual and societal burden of chronic pain in Europe: The case for strategic prioritisation and action to improve knowledge and availability of care. *BMC Public Health, 12,* 1229.

Bringsvor, H. B., Skaug, K., Langeland, E., Oftedal, B. F., Assmuss, J., Gundersen, D., Osborne, R. H., & Bentsen, S. B. (2018). Symptom burden and self-management in persons with chronic obstructive pulmonary disease. *International Journal of COPD, 13,* 365–373.

British Medical Association. (2019). *Prevention before cure: Prioritising population health.* London: British Medical Association.

British Pain Society. (2013). *Guidelines for pain management programmes for adults: An evidence-based review prepared on behalf of the British Pain Society.* London: The British Pain Society.

British Pain Society. Retrieved November 25, 2019, from https://www.british-painsociety.org/people-with-pain/frequently-asked-questions/#what-is-pain.

British Pain Society Website. Retrieved from https://www.britishpainsociety.org/about/what-is-pain/

Buck, D. (2018). Blog post: Prevention is better than cure, except when it comes to paying for it. Retrieved December 2, 2019, from https://www.kingsfund.org.uk/blog/2018/11/prevention-better-cure-except-when-it-comes-paying-it

Callahan, C. M. (2001). Quality improvement research on late life depression in primary care. *Medical Care, 39*(8), 772–784.

Campbell, R., Evans, M., Tucker, M., Quilty, B., Dieppe, P., & Donovan, J. L. (2001). Why don't patients do their exercises? Understanding non-compliance with physiotherapy in patients with osteoarthritis of the knee. *Journal of Epidemiology and Community Health, 55,* 131–138.

Carroll, L. J., Rother, J. P., & Ozegovic, D. (2013). What does coping mean to the worker with pain-related disability. *Disability and Rehabilitation, 35*(14), 1182–1190.

Chesanow, N. (2015). The art of handling 'difficult' patients. *Medscape*, February 23. Retrieved November 25, 2019, from https://www.medscape.com/viewarticle/838283.

Chronic Pain Policy Coalition. (2015). *The hidden suffering of chronic pain.* London: Chronic Pain Policy Coalition.

Clark, W. C., Yang, J. C., Tsui, S. L., Ng, K. F., & Clark, S. B. (2002). Unidimensional pain rating scales: A multidimensional affect and pain survey (MAPS) analysis of what they really measure. *Pain, 98,* 241–247.

Code of Practice for Residential Estate Agents. Retrieved November 25, 2019, from https://www.tpos.co.uk/codes-of-practice

Coulter, A., Roberts, S., & Dixon, A. (2013). *Delivering better services for people with long-term-conditions: Building the house of care.* London: The King's Fund.

Craig, K. D. (2009). The social communication model of pain. *Canadian Psychology, 50*(1), 22–32.

Crosby, C. (2016). *A body undone: Living on after great pain.* New York: New York University Press.

CSPMS UK. (2015). *Core standards for pain management in the UK.* London: Faculty of Pain Medicine.

Davies, M. (2013). Managing challenging interactions with patients. *BMJ, 347,* f4673. https://doi.org/10.1136/bmj.f4673.

De Ruddere, L., Goubert, L., Prkachin, K. M., Stevens, M. L. A., Van Ryckeghem, D. M. L., & Crombez, G. (2011). When you dislike patients, pain is taken less seriously. *Pain, 152*(10), 2342–2347.

De Ruddere, L., Goubert, L., Stevens, M., Williams, A. C. d. C., & Crombez, G. (2013). Discounting pain in the absence of medical evidence is explained by negative evaluation of the patient. *Pain, 154*(5), 669–676.

De Ruddere, L., Goubert, L., Stevens, M. A. L., Deveugele, M., Craig, K. D., & Crombez, G. (2014). Health care professionals' reactions to patient pain: Impact of knowledge about medical evidence and psychosocial influences. *The Journal of Pain, 15*(3), 262–270.

De Ruddere, L., Goubert, L., Vervoort, T., Prkachin, K. M., & Crombez, G. (2012). We discount the pain of others when pain has no medical explanation. *The Journal of Pain, 13*(12), 1198–1205.

Department of Health. (2006). *Supporting people with long term conditions to self-care: A guide to developing local strategies and good practice.* London: Department of Health.

Department of Health. (2009). *Your Health, your way. A guide to long term conditions and self-care.* London: Department of Health.

Department of Health & Social Care (DHSC). (2018). *Prevention is better than cure: Our vision to help you live well for longer.* London: Department of Health and Social Care, Gov.uk.

Department of Health & Social Care (DHSC). (2018). *Framework agreement between the Department of Health & Social Care and the National Institute for Health and Care Excellence*. London: DHSC, NICE.

Department of Health & Social Care (DHSC). (2019). *The government's 2019–20 accountability framework with NHS England and NHS improvement*. London: DHSC.

Dickson, A., Ward, R., O'Brien, G., Allen, D., & O'Carroll, R. (2011). Difficulties adjusting to post-discharge life following a spinal cord injury: An interpretative phenomenological analysis. *Psychology, Health and Medicine, 16*(4), 463–474.

Donaldson, L. (2008). *150 years of the annual report of the Chief Medical Officer: On the state of public health 2018*. London: Department of Health.

Donovan, J. L., & Blake, D. R. (2000). Qualitative study of interpretation of reassurance among patients attending rheumatology clinics: "Just a touch of arthritis, doctor?". *BMJ, 320*, 541–544.

Dow, C. M., Roche, P. A., & Ziebland, S. (2012). Talk of frustration in the narratives of people with chronic pain. *Chronic Illness, 8*(3), 176–191.

Dunahoo, C. L., Hobfoll, S. E., Monnier, J., Hulsizer, M. R., & Johnson, R. (1998). There's more to rugged individualism in coping. Part 1: Even the Lone Ranger had Tonto. *Anxiety, Stress, Coping: An International Journal, 11*(2), 137–165.

Dures, E., Fraser, I., Almeida, C., Peterson, A., Caesley, J., Pollock, J., Ambler, N., Morris, M., & Hewlett, S. (2016). Patients' perspectives on the psychological impact of inflammatory arthritis and meeting the associated support needs: Open-ended responses in a multi-centre survey. *Musculoskeletal Care, 15*, 175–185.

Dwarswaard, J., Bakker, E. J. M., van Staa, A., & Boeje, H. (2015). Self-management support from the perspective of patients with a chronic condition: A thematic synthesis of qualitative studies. *Health Expectations, 19*, 194–208.

Eaton, L. H., Langford, D. J., Meins, A. R., Rue, T., Tauben, D. J., & Doorenbos, A. Z. (2018). Use of self-management interventions for chronic pain management: A comparison between rural and non-rural residents. *Pain Management Nursing, 19*(1), 8–13.

Eccleston, C., Morley, S. J., & Williams, A. C. d. C. (2013). Psychological approaches to chronic pain management: Evidence and challenges. *British Journal of Anaesthesia, 111*(1), 59–63.

Eccleston, C., Williams, A. C. D. C., & Rogers, W. S. (1997). Patients' and professionals' understandings of the causes of chronic pain: Blame, responsibility and identity protection. *Social Science and Medicine, 45*(5), 699–709.

Effing, T. W., Vercoulen, J. H., Bourbeau, J., Trappenburg, J., Lenferink, A., Cafarella, P., et al. (2016). Definition of a COPD self-management intervention: International Expert Group consensus. *European Respiratory Journal, 48*, 46–54.

Entwistle, V. A., Cribb, A., & Owens, J. (2018a). Why health and social care support for people with long-term conditions should be oriented towards enabling them to live well. *Health Care Analysis, 26*, 48–65.

Entwistle, V. A., Cribb, A., Watt, I. S., Skea, Z. C., Owens, J., Morgan, H. M., & Christmas, S. (2018b). "The more you know, the more you realise it is really challenging to do": Tensions and uncertainties in person-centred support for people with long-term conditions. *Patient Education and Counseling, 101*, 1460–1467.

Fayaz, A., Croft, P., Langford, R. M., Donaldson, L. J., & Jones, G. T. (2016). Prevalence of chronic pain in the UK: A systematic review and meta-analysis of population studies. *BMJ Open, 6*, e010364. https://doi.org/10.1136/bmjopen-2015-010364.

Finlay, K. A., & Elander, J. (2016). Reflecting the transition from pain management services to chronic pain support group attendance: An interpretative phenomenological analysis. *British Journal of Health Psychology, 21*, 660–676.

Folkman, S., & Moskowitz, J. T. (2004). Coping: Pitfalls and promise. *Annual Review of Psychology, 55*, 745–774.

Fonte, D., Lagouanelle-Simeon, M. C., & Apostolidis, T. (2017). "Behave like a responsible adult"—Relation between social identity and psychosocial skills at stake in self-management of a chronic disease. *Self and Identity*. https://doi.org/10.1080/15298868.2017.1371636.

Francis, H., Carryer, J., & Wilkinson, J. (2018). Patient expertise: Contested territory in the realm of long-term condition care. *Chronic Illness, 15*(3), 197–209.

Frayne, D. (2019). *The work cure: Critical essays on work and wellness*. Monmouth: PCCS Books.

Fu, Y., Yu, G., McNichol, E., Marczewski, K., & Closs, S. J. (2018). The association between patient-professional partnerships and self-management of chronic back pain: A mixed methods study. *European Journal of Pain, 22*(7), 1229–1244.

Galasinski, D. (2017). Difficult patients. Retrieved November 25, 2019, from http://dariuszgalasinski.com/2017/08/12/difficult-patients/

Gallant, M. P. (2003). The influence of social support on chronic illness self-management: A review and directions for research. *Health Education and Behaviour, 30*, 170–195.

Gauntlett-Gilbert, J., Rodham, K., Jordan, A., & Brook, P. (2015). Emergency Department staff attitudes toward people presenting in chronic pain: A qualitative study. *Pain Medicine., 16*(11), 2065–2074.

Gilbert, P. (2000). The relationship of shame, social anxiety and depression: The role of the evaluation of social rank. *Clinical Psychology and Psychotherapy, 7*, 174–189.

Gilbert, P., Pehl, J., & Allan, S. (1994). The phenomenology of shame and guilt: An empirical investigation. *British Journal of Medical Psychology, 67*, 23–36.

Glenton, C. (2003). Chronic back pain sufferers—striving for the sick role. *Social Science and Medicine, 57,* 2243–2252.

Goodwin, N., Curry, N., Naylor, C., Ross, S., & Duldig, W. (2010). *Managing people with long-term conditions.* London: King's Fund.

Grady, P. A., & Gough, R. N. (2014). Self-management: A comprehensive approach to the management of chronic conditions. *Framing Health Matters, 104*(8), e25–e31.

Granger, B., Sandelowski, M., Tahshjain, H., Swedberg, K., & Ekman, I. (2009). A qualitative descriptive study of the work of adherence to a chronic heart failure regimen: Patient and physician perspectives. *Journal of Cardiovascular Nursing, 24*(4), 308–315.

Greaves, L. (2015). The meanings of smoking to women and their implications for cessation. *International Journal of Environmental Research and Public Health., 12*(2), 1449–1465.

Greenhalgh, T., & Papoutsi, C. (2018). Studying complexity in health services research: Desperately seeking an overdue paradigm shift. *BMC Medicine, 16,* 95. https://doi.org/10.1186/s12916-01801089-4.

Health Foundation. (2011). *Helping people help themselves: A review of the evidence considering whether it is worthwhile to support self-management.* London: The Health Foundation.

Health Foundation. (2015). *A practical guide to self-management support: Key components for successful implementation.* London: The Health Foundation.

Hinder, S., & Greenhalgh, T. (2012). "This does my head in": Ethnographic study of self-management by people with diabetes. *BMC Health Services Research, 12,* 83.

Hochschild, A. R. (1979). Emotion work, feeling rules, and social structure. *American Journal of Sociology, 85*(3), 551–575.

Hughes, M. (2017). Strategies for helping chronic pain patients. *BC Psychologists, 6*(3) (Summer), 18–20.

Hush, J. M., Refshauge, K. M., Sullivan, G., De Souza, L., & McCauley, J. H. (2010). Do numerical rating scales and the Roland-Morris disability questionnaire capture changes that are meaningful to patients with persistent back pain? *Clinical Rehabilitation, 24,* 648–657.

IASP. Retrieved November 25, 2019, from https://www.iasp-pain.org/Education/Content.aspx?ItemNumber=1698.

Jensen, M. P., Johnson, L. E., Gertz, K. J., Galer, B. S., & Gammaitoni, A. R. (2013). The words patients use to describe chronic pain: Implications for measuring pain quality. *Pain, 154,* 2722–2728.

Keene, D. E., Guo, M., & Murillo, S. (2018). That wasn't really a place to worry about diabetes: Housing access and diabetes self-management among low income adults. *Social Science and Medicine, 197,* 71–77.

Kelly, M. P., & Barker, M. (2016). Why is changing health-related behaviour so difficult? *Public Health, 136,* 109–116.

Kenning, C., Fisher, L., Bee, P., Bower, P., & Coventry, P. (2013). Primary care practitioner and patient understanding of the concepts of multimorbidity and self-management: A qualitative study. *SAGE Open Medicine, 1.* https://doi. org/10.1177/2050312113510001.

Kenny, D. T. (2004). Constructions of chronic pain in doctor-patient relationships: Bridging the communication chasm. *Patient Education and Counselling, 52,* 297–305.

Kenny, D. T., Trevorrow, T., Heard, R., & Faunce, G. (2006). Communicating pain: Do people share an understanding of the meaning of pain descriptors? *Australian Psychologist, 41*(3), 213–218.

Kinderman, P. (2019). *A manifesto for mental health: Why we need a revolution in mental health care.* Palgrave Macmillan.

King, A., & Hoppe, R. B. (2013). "Best practice" for patient-centred communication: A narrative review. *Journal of Graduate Medical Education, 5,* 385–393. https://doi.org/10.4300/JGME-D-13-00072./.

Koekkoek, B., Hutschemaekers, G., Meijel, B. V., & Shcene, A. (2011). How do patients come to be seen as 'difficult'?: A mixed-methods study in community mental health care. *Social Science and Medicine, 72,* 5040512.

Kohut, S. A., Stinson, J., Forgeron, P., Wyk, M. V., Harris, L., & Luca, S. (2018). A qualitative content analysis of peer mentoring video calls in adolescents with chronic illness. *Journal of Health Psychology, 23*(6), 788–789.

Kool, M., van Middendorp, H., Boeije, H. R., & Geenen, R. (2009). Understanding the lack of understanding: Invalidation from the perspective of the patient with Fibromyalgia. *Arthritis & Rheumatism, 61*(12), 1650–1656.

Kotarba, J. A. (1983). *Chronic pain: Its social dimensions.* London: Sage.

Kristjansdottir, O. B., Stenberg, U., Mirkovic, J., Krogseth, T., Ljosa, T. M., Stange, K. C., & Ruland, C. M. (2018). Personal strengths reported by people with chronic illness: A qualitative study. *Health Expectations, 21*(4), 787–795.

Kropotkin, P. (1913). Retrieved December 14, 2019, from https://theanarchistlibrary.org/library/petr-kropotkin-prisons-universities-of-crime

Kugelmann, R. (1997). The psychology and management of pain. *Theory and Psychology, 7,* 43–65.

Lazarus, R. S., & Folkman, S. (1984). *Stress appraisal and coping.* New York: Springer.

Le Vasseur, J. J. (2003). The problem of bracketing in phenomenology. *Qualitative Health Research, 13,* 408–420.

Lennox Thompson, B. (2019). Living well with chronic pain: A classical grounded theory. *Disability and Rehabilitation.* https://doi.org/10.1080/0963828 8.2018.1517195.

Loftus, S. (2011). Pain and its metaphors: A dialogical approach. *Journal of Medical Humanities, 31,* 213–230.

Lorig, K. R., & Holman, H. R. (2003). Self-management education: History, definition, outcomes and mechanisms. *Annals of Behavioral Medicine, 26*(1), 1–7.

Mackay, H. (2018). Wheelchair shortage: "I had to carry my son after he broke his leg". *BBC News Website,* July 27. Retrieved November 18, 2019, from https://www.bbc.co.uk/news/uk-44964130

MacLeod, A. D. (2004). Shell shock, Gordon Holmes and the Great War. *Journal of the Royal Society of Medicine, 97,* 86–89.

Marshall, L. (2016). The economic case for preventing ill health. Blog post, July 25. Retrieved December 2, 2019, from https://www.health.org.uk/blogs/the-economic-case-for-preventing-ill-health

Martin, F., Camfield, L., Rodham, K., Kliempt, P., & Ruta, D. (2007). 12 Years' experience with the Patient Generated Index (PGI) of Quality of Life: A graded structured review. *Quality of Life Research, 16,* 705–715.

Masupe, T. K., Ndayi, K., Tsolekile, L., Delobelle, P., & Puoane, T. (2018). Redefining diabetes and the concept of self-management from a patient's perspective: Implications for disease risk-factor management. *Health Education Research, 33*(1), 40–54.

McCaffery, M. (1968). *Nursing practice theories related to cognition, bodily pain, and man- environment interactions.* Los Angeles: University of California at Los Angeles Students' Store.

Melzack, R. (1975). The McGill Pain Questionnaire: Major properties and scoring methods. *Pain, 1,* 277–299.

Melzack, R. (2005). The McGill Pain Questionnaire: From description to measurement. *Anesthesiology, 103,* 199–202.

Melzack, R., & Torgerson, W. S. (1971). On the language of pain. *Anesthesiology, 34,* 50–59.

Michie, S., & Abraham, C. (2008). Advancing the science of behaviour change techniques used in interventions. *Health Psychology, 27*(3), 379–387.

Michie, S., Atkins, L., & West, R. (2014). *The behaviour change wheel: A guide to designing interventions.* London: Silverback Publishing.

Moore, P. Pain Toolkit Website. Retrieved from https://www.paintoolkit.org/

Moore, A. J., Richardson, J. C., Bernard, M., & Sim, J. (2018). Interpreting intracorporeal landscapes: How patients visualise pathophysiology and utilize medical images in their understanding of chronic musculoskeletal illness. *Disability and Rehabilitation.* https://doi.org/10.1080/0963828 8.2018.1443162.

Morgan, H. M., Entwistle, V. A., Cribb, A., Christmas, S., Owens, J., Skea, Z. C., & Watt, I. S. (2016). We need to talk about purpose: A critical interpretive synthesis of health and social care professionals' approaches to self-management for people with long-term conditions. *Health Expectations, 20,* 243–259.

Moseley, G. L., & Butler, D. S. (2015). Fifteen years of explaining pain: The past, present and future. *The Journal of Pain, 16*(9), 807–813.

Moss-Morris, R. (2013). Adjusting to chronic illness: Time for a unified theory. *British Journal of Health Psychology, 18,* 681–686.

Murray, M. (2018). The pre-history of health psychology in the United Kingdom: From natural science and psychoanalysis to social science, social cognition and beyond. *Journal of Health Psychology, 23*(3), 472–491.

Murray, R. (2019). The NHS long-term plan: Five things you need to know. Retrieved from https://www.kingsfund.org.uk/blog/2019/01/nhs-long-term-plan

National Pain Audit. (2013). *National Pain Audit Final Report, 2010–2012.* London: The British Pain Society.

National Primary Care Network. (2017). *Improving accountability in the provision of new models of care.* London: National Association of Primary Care.

Navarro, K., Wainwright, E., Rodham, K., & Jordan, A. (2018). Parenting people with complex regional pain syndrome: An analysis of the process of parental online communication. *Pain Reports, 3,* e681.

Naylor, C., Imison, C., Smithson, R., Buck, D., Goodwin, N., Ross, S., Sonola, L., Tian, Y., & Curry, N. (2015). Transforming our healthcare system: Ten Priorities for commissioners. Retrieved from https://www.kingsfund.org.uk/publications/articles/transforming-our-health-care-system-ten-priorities-commissioners

NHS. (2006). *Supporting people with long term conditions to self-care.* London: Department of Health.

NHS. (2019). Long term plan. Retrieved from https://www.longterm-plan.nhs.uk/

NICE. (2011). *Diabetes in adults: quality standard (QS6).* London: National Institute for Health and Clinical Excellence.

NICE. (2012). *Patient experience in adult NHS services: Improving the experience of care for people using adult NHS services.* London: NICE.

NICE Pain Guidelines. Retrieved from https://www.nice.org.uk/guidance/indevelopment/gid-ng10069/documents

Nøst, T. H., Steinsbekk, A., Bratas, O., & Grønning, K. (2018). Short-term effect of a chronic pain self-management intervention delivered by an easily accessible primary healthcare service: A randomised controlled trial. *BMJ Open, 8,* e023017.

Osborn, M., & Smith, J. A. (1998). The personal experience of chronic benign lower back pain: An Interpretative phenomenological analysis. *British Journal of Health Psychology, 3,* 65–83.

Osborne, R. H., Elsworth, G. R., & Whitfield, K. (2007). The Health Education Impact Questionnaire (heiQ): An outcomes and evaluation measure for patient education and self-management interventions for people with chronic conditions. *Patient Education and Counselling, 66*(2), 192–201.

Oxford Library of Words and Phrases. (1993). *Volume 1: The concise Oxford dictionary of quotations.* London: BCA.

Packer, T. L., Fracini, A., Audulv, A., Alizadeh, N., Gaal, B. G. I. V., Warner, G., & Kephart, G. (2018). What we know about the purpose, theoretical foundation, scope and dimensionality of existing self-management measurement tools: A scoping review. *Patient Education and Counseling, 101*(4), 579–595.

Padilha, J. M., Sousa, P. A. F., & Pereira, F. M. S. (2017). Nursing clinical practice changes to improve self-management in chronic obstructive pulmonary disease. *International Nursing Review, 65*(1), 122–130.

Paige, S. R., Stellefson, M., & Singh, B. (2016). Patient perspectives on factors associated with enrolment and retention in chronic disease self-management programs: A systematic review. *Patient Intelligence, 8, 21–37.*

Pain Concern. (2019). Self-management navigator tool. Retrieved January 6, 2020, from http://painconcern.org.uk/navigator-tool/

Pickles, K., Eassey, D., Reddel, H. K., Locock, L., Kirkpatrick, S., & Smith, L. (2018). "This illness diminishes me. What it does it like theft": A qualitative meta-synthesis of people's experiences of living with asthma. *Health Expectations, 21,* 23–40.

Potter, C. M., Kelly, L., Hunter, C., Fitzpatrick, R., & Peters, M. (2018). The context of coping: A qualitative exploration of underlying inequalities that influence health services support for people living with long term conditions. *Sociology of Health & Illness, 40*(1), 130–145.

Reidy, C., Kennedy, A., Pope, C., Ballinger, C., Vassilev, I., & Rogers, A. (2016). Commissioning self-management support for people with long-term conditions: An exploration of commissioning aspirations and processes. *BMJ Open, 6,* e010853.

Reynolds, R., Dennis, S., Hasan, I., Slewa, J., Chen, W., Tian, D., Bobba, S., & Zwar, N. (2018). A systematic review of chronic disease management interventions in primary care. *BMC Family Practice, 19,* 11. https://doi.org/10.1186/s12875-017-0692-3.

Rhodes, E. (2017). UN report points to power imbalances. *The Psychologist.* Retrieved December 14, 2019, from https://thepsychologist.bps.org.uk/volume-30/september-2017/un-report-points-power-imbalances.

Rochman, D. L. (1998). Students' knowledge of pain: A survey of four schools. *Occupational Therapy International, 5*(2), 140–154.

Rodham, K. (2015). *Learning to cope with CRPS/RSD: Putting life first and pain second.* London: Singing Dragon.

Rodham, K. (2018a). *The making of a crazy cat lady.* Lulu Publishers.

Rodham, K. (2018b). CRPS and self-management. In *CRPS UK Conference*, October 20, 2018, Bath.

Rodham, K., Boxell, E., McCabe, C., Cockburn, M., & Waller, E. (2012). Transitioning from a hospital rehabilitation programme to home: Exploring the experiences of people with Complex Regional Pain Syndrome. *Psychology and Health, 27*(10), 1150–1165.

Rodham, K., Gavin, J., Coulson, N., & Watts, L. (2015). Co-creation of information leaflets to meet the support needs of people living with Complex Regional Pain Syndrome (CRPS) through innovative use of wiki technology. *Informatics for Health and Social Care, 41*(3), 325–339.

Royal College of Obstetricians and Gynaecologists. (2019). Retrieved December 23, 2019, from https://www.rcog.org.uk/better-for-women/.

Russell, S., Ogunbayo, O. J., Newham, J. J., Heslop-Marshall, K., Netts, P., Hanratty, B., Beyer, F., & Kaner, E. (2018). Qualitative systematic review of barriers and facilitators to self-management of chronic pulmonary disease: Views of patients and healthcare professionals. *Primary Care Respiratory Medicine, 2*. https://doi.org/10.1038/s41533-017-0069-2.

Sadler, E., Wolfe, C. D. A., Jones, F., & McKevitt, C. (2017). Exploring stroke survivors' and physiotherapists' views of self-management after stroke: A qualitative study in the UK. *BMJ Open, 7*, e011631.

Salisbury, H. (2019). Helen Salisbury: The informed patient. *BMJ, 364*, l638.

Salmon, P., Mendick, N., & Young, B. (2011). Integrative qualitative communication analysis of consultation and patient and practitioner perspectives: Towards a theory of authentic caring in clinical relationships. *Patient Education and Counseling, 82*, 448–454.

Seers, T., Derry, S., Seers, K., & Moore, R. A. (2018). Professionals underestimate patients' pain: A comprehensive review. *Pain, 159*(5), 811–815.

Senior, T. (2018). How chronic diseases thrive. *British Journal of General Practice.* https://doi.org/10.3399/bjgp18X698237.

Shaikh, M., & Hapidou, E. G. (2018). Factors involved in patients' perceptions of self-improvement after chronic pain treatment. *Canadian Journal of Pain, 2*(1), 145–157.

Shim, J. K. (2010). Cultural health capital: A theoretical approach to understanding health care interactions and the dynamics of unequal treatment. *Journal of Health and Social Behaviour, 51*(1), 1–15.

Singleton, W. T. (1964). A preliminary study of a Capstan Lathe. *International Journal of Production Research, 3*(3), 213.

Slightam, C. A., Brandt, K., Jenchura, E. C., Lewis, E. T., Asch, S. M., & Zulman, D. M. (2018). "I had to change so much in my life to live with my new limitations": Multimorbid patients' descriptions of their most bothersome chronic conditions. *Chronic Illness, 14*(1), 13–24.

Smith, J. A., & Osborn, M. (2007). Pain as an assault on the self: An interpretative phenomenological analysis of the psychological impact of chronic benign low back pain. *Psychology and Health, 22*(5), 517–534.

Snow, R., Humphrey, C., & Sandall, J. (2013). What happens when patients know more than their doctors? Experiences of heath interactions after diabetes patient education: A qualitative patient-led study. *BMJ Open, 3*, e003583.

SNRPMP. (2015). Retrieved from https://www.snrpmp.scot.nhs.uk/

Sointu, E. (2017). 'Good' patient/'bad' patient: Clinical learning and the entrenching of inequality. *Sociology of Health and Illness, 39*(1), 63–77.

Sullivan, M. J. L. (2012). The communal coping model of pain catastrophising: Clinical and research implications. *Canadian Psychology, 53*(1), 32–41.

Tod, A. M. (2003). Barriers to smoking cessation in pregnancy: A qualitative study. *British Journal of Community Nursing., 8*, 56–64.

Todd, A., Akhter, N., Cairns, J. M., Kasim, A., Walton, N., Ellison, A., Chazot, P., Eldabe, S., & Bambra, C. (2018). The pain divide: A cross-sectional analysis of chronic pain prevalence, pain intensity and opioid utilisation in England. *BMJ Open, 8*, e023391. https://doi.org/10.1136/b,jopen-2018-023391.

Turk, D. C., & Okifuji, A. (1999). Psychological factors in chronic pain: Evolution and revolution. *Journal of Consulting and Clinical Psychology, 70*(3), 678–690.

Vermeer, A., & Wenting, B. (2016). *Self-management: How does it work?* Amsterdam: Reed Business Information.

Westland, H., Schröder, C. D., Wit, J., Frings, J., Trappenburg, J. C. A., & Schuurmans, M. J. (2018). Self-management support in routine primary care by nurses. *British Journal of Health Psychology, 23*, 88–107.

White, K., Issac, M. S. M., Kamoun, C., Leygues, J., & Cohn, S. (2018). The THRIVE model: A framework and review of internal and external predictors of coping with chronic illness. *Health Psychology Open*, Jul-Dec, 1–14. https://doi.org/10.1177/2055102918793552.

Wilkinson, R., & Marmot, M. (Eds.). (2003). *Social determinants of health: The solid facts*. World Health Organisation.

Williams, A. C. D. C., Davies, H. T. O., & Chadury, Y. (2000). Simple pain rating scales hide complex idiosyncratic meanings. *Pain, 85*, 457–463.

Yorkston, K. M., Johnson, K., Boesflug, E., Skala, J., & Amtmann, D. (2010). Communicating about the experience of pain and fatigue in disability. *Quality of Life Research, 19*, 243–251.

Youngson, R. (2008). Disabled doctoring: How can we rehabilitate the medical profession? *Alan Clarke Memorial Lecture*, November 27, at the Australian and New Zealand Spinal Cord Society Conference, Christchurch New Zealand. Retrieved December 2, 2019, from https://docplayer.net/161017698-Disabled-doctoring-how-can-we-rehabilitate-the-medical-profession.html.

Youngson, R. (2012). *Time to care: How to love your patients and your job*. New Zealand: Rebelheart Publishers.

INDEX

© The Author(s) 2020
K. Rodham, *Self-Management for Persistent Pain*,
https://doi.org/10.1007/978-3-030-48969-4